Men's Health

THE
CommonSense
APPROACH

GW00357178

The CommonSense Approach Series

This series of self-help guides from Newleaf provides practical and sound ways to deal with many of life's common complaints.

Each book in the series is written for the layperson, and adopts a commonsense approach to the many questions surrounding a particular topic. It explains what the complaint is, how and why it occurs, and what can be done about it. It includes advice on helping ourselves, and information on where to go for further help. It encourages us to take responsibility for our own health, to be sensible and not always to rely on medical intervention for every ill.

Men's Health

THE
CommonSense
APPROACH

Joe Armstrong

Newleaf

Newleaf

an imprint of
Gill & Macmillan Ltd
Goldenbridge
Dublin 8
with associated companies throughout the world
www.gillmacmillan.ie
© Joe Armstrong 1999
0 7171 2802 4
Index compiled by Helen Litton
Design by Identikit Design Consultants, Dublin
Print origination by Carole Lynch
Printed by ColourBooks Ltd, Dublin

This book is typeset in Revivial565 9.5pt on 15pt.

A CIP catalogue record for this book is available
from the British Library.

1 3 5 4 2

Contents

Foreword

Many years ago I went up to a man and said, 'Do you know that four times as many men die from prostate cancer than women die from cervical cancer?' He looked at me as if I had just landed from another planet. 'What', he replied with a look we once called old-fashioned, 'has it go to do with being prostrate?'

Those were the days before Joe Armstrong began successfully to highlight the anomaly in Irish men's health. Being at least five years ahead of his time can be tricky: men's health issues were once not PC topics for conversation, yet Joe has been writing about it before people realised that being a man can seriously damage your health.

Like any pioneer, others followed, and now there is an increasing number of books on the subject. Most of them are written by people with only an academic interest which is why this book is so refreshingly welcome.

Men see their doctor half as often as do women and when they finally drag themselves into the surgery it is invariably later in the course of any disease. So us men need a *CommonSense Approach* if we are to redress the balance leaving us dying six years earlier than those non-members of the prostrate owners' club.

It's all very well pointing out the problem: getting men to do something about it is not so easy and there is no shortage of well-meaning pontifications lying unread in bookshops. I suspect this up-to-date, factually accurate, informative and down-to-earth book will spend less time on shelves and more time doing the job it is so well designed to do: improving men's health.

Having a book in the house which is enjoyable to read yet supplies no shortage of F-Me-Facts (Goodness me, I never knew that before) makes sense. Joe Armstrong makes common sense of men's health.

Dr Ian Banks
Chair, All-Ireland Men's Health Forum
Chair, UK Men's Health Forum
British Medical Association Spokesman on men's health issues
Medical editor, *Men's Health Magazine*

Acknowledgments

I want to thank Caroline Walsh, Literary Editor at *The Irish Times*, who, as Features Editor, invited me to write the 'Man Alive' men's health column, which, in turn, has led to this book. Thank you, too, to readers, male and female, who encouraged me to develop that column into this more lasting book form. Although some of the chapters here are close to the original *Irish Times* column, everything has been completely reviewed, updated and reworked, while many new topics and issues are here explored by this writer for the first time.

Thank you to the many health professionals, academics and friends, most of whom are named in these pages, who generously permitted their brains to be picked for this book. Without them, neither 'Man Alive' nor *Men's Health — The CommonSense Approach* could have come into being.

Finally, and most of all, I want to thank my dear and long-suffering wife, Ruth, and our young children, John and Sarah, for their patient, supportive and playful presence during the adventure of writing this book.

While the author has made every effort to ensure that the information contained in this book is accurate, it should not be regarded as an alternative to professional medical advice. Readers should consult their general practitioners or physicians if they are concerned about aspects of their own health, and before embarking on any course of treatment. Neither the author, nor the publishers, can accept responsibility for any health problem resulting from using, or discontinuing, any of the drugs described here, or the self-help methods described.

Introduction

Men's health is in dire straits . . .

◆ Men die about six years younger than women. On average, Irish males can expect to live to 72.6 years; British men live to 73.5; Swedish men make it to 75.1; while Japanese men die at 76.6 years.

◆ In Ireland and the UK, nearly half of all men die from heart disease and related conditions like stroke. Heart disease kills at least one in every three men in the Western World, while high blood pressure (Chapter 6) affects one in five. Men having a heart attack often haven't a clue what to do. Some go for a walk to see if it will go away — the very opposite to what they should do (see Chapter 4).

◆ Women, during their childbearing years, have greater protection than men against heart disease because of estrogen and progesterone in their bodies.

◆ Up to 30 per cent of men in their 50s and up to 70 per cent of men in their 70s have prostate cancer (Chapter 3). As many as one in 32 males develop it, which makes prostate cancer in men almost as common as breast cancer in women.

◆ Almost five times as many men die from cancer of the prostate as the number of women who die from cervical cancer; yet prostatic cancer is much less researched.

◆ As many as a quarter of men who live to 80 will require a prostatectomy, the surgical removal of a portion of the prostate.

- Some 14 per cent of men in their 40s have symptoms of benign prostatic hyperplasia (BPH), experienced as discomfort or pain in passing urine (Chapter 3); as do 24 per cent of men in their 50s and 40 per cent of men in their 60s. Many needlessly suffer in silence when it could be investigated and treated.

- Testicular cancer (Chapter 2) is the commonest form of cancer in young men aged 15 to 44. One in every 273 men will develop it. Some needlessly die from it each year because of failure to detect it in time.

- One in three men gets cancer and one in four dies from it.

- Melanoma kills more men than women — even though more women get it than men.

- Three times as many men die in car crashes as women, often due to alcohol or speeding.

- Men are more likely to be killed in workplace accidents than women, and they are more likely to earn their living in dangerous occupations like construction, mining or fishing.

- Males suffer greater injuries as a result of contact sports than females.

- Most alcoholics, drug addicts and patients in mental hospitals are male.

- Men smoke themselves to an early grave. About 11 men die every day in Ireland due to smoking, compared to 6.8 smoking-related female fatalities a day. Some 219 men and 113 women die every day in the UK due to smoking.

- Most sexually transmitted diseases have a higher incidence rate among men than women (Chapter 19).

- Men also suffer from conditions mistakenly assumed only to affect women. Men get breast cancer, osteoporosis (the bone-wasting disease) and the eating disorders anorexia and bulimia nervosa (Chapter 5).

- The vast majority of people who take their own lives are male (Chapter 13). Although depression (Chapter 12) is twice as high in women, 4.5 times as many men as women take their own lives. Suicide is a major cause of death among males aged 15 to 24. Women appear to ask for help. Men tend not to.

◆ A lot of men are emotionally illiterate and, in particular, have difficulties with anger (Chapter 8), fear (Chapter 9) and jealousy (Chapter 10). To identify and own an authentic, self-originating feeling can be a giant leap forward for some men.

◆ Many men, young and old, have inadequate coping skills in dealing with critical losses like bereavement, separation, divorce, redundancy or retirement (Chapter 11).

◆ It is estimated that 140 million men worldwide suffer from impotence. Some 40 per cent of men over the age of 40 suffer from it for extended periods. Viagra, the impotence pill, became the fastest-selling new drug in the US in 1998, with some 10,000 prescriptions for it being written every day (Chapter 15).

◆ Ten per cent of the male population is now regarded as subfertile, while controversial studies have suggested that male infertility is increasing at an alarming rate (Chapter 16).

◆ Male rape is seldom discussed but regularly occurs. In Ireland alone, at least one male is raped every month, by strangers, acquaintances, relatives, family friends, lodgers, prison inmates, ministers of religion and employers (Chapter 18).

◆ Men need to know about the wide range of sexually transmitted diseases to reduce the likelihood of exposing themselves, or their partners, to ill-health or an untimely death (Chapter 19).

◆ Men are more likely than women to suffer from damage to their health due to shift-work. Many men have conditions which — often unknown to them — make it unwise for them to do night work (see Chapter 20). Meanwhile, five times as many men as women need treatment for snoring.

◆ Men tend to suffer from more severe acne than women. Up to 80 per cent of adolescent males get acne, while up to five per cent of men in their 20s and 30s have it. Some men are driven to suicide because of it (Chapter 23).

◆ Even in the womb, male fatality rates are disproportionately high. Most miscarried foetuses are male.

◆ Most babies born with congenital abnormalities are boys.

◆ The mortality rate in the first year of life is higher for males than for females.

Men — especially young men — often act as though they will live for ever. They act as if they don't need to look after their health. Or they know they should but, like Saint Augustine, say 'Not yet.'

Some men, who in other spheres are responsible, can be fatalistic when it comes to their health. While they adopt an intelligent, strategic approach to their finances, career development, car maintenance or to training for their favourite sport, they can regress to near-infantile fatalism when it comes to their health: 'When your time's up, your time's up.' 'No point being the healthiest corpse in the cemetery.' Or the crass 'So what if it's bad for you!'

Men are much less likely than women to consult a doctor but are much more likely to be rushed to hospital with a heart attack or stroke.

This book aims to alert men, and those close to them, about the need to look after their health. It is also for mothers, wives and the partners of the male of the species.

Managing men's health is more important than managing our shekels, BMW or the great career plan. We need information about it. We need to learn from women how to prevent illness rather than be struck by sickness or death too soon down the road. Our bodies are our tickets to staying a little longer on this planet. Let's take care of them. Gentlemen — young and old — this is your wake-up call.

PART I

Men's Bodies

CHAPTER 1

The Penis

The penis is an amazing organ. From the moment a human is born, he or she is, to a large extent, defined by the penis — or its absence.

Your name, the first clothes you wear (and whether you progress to an Armani suit or a revealing Lainey Keogh number), the unspoken expectations laid upon you from birth, the family roles you play, the schools you attend, the sexual expectations placed upon you, your choice of career, the roles that are opened or denied to you by your family, faith or fatherland — all these are shaped to a significant degree by your gender or sex.

Men, in the main, don't tend to be named Veronica. Boys don't usually wear dresses. Boy-toddlers who kiss other little boys can raise an adult's eyebrow. Rough-playing little girls soon get dubbed 'tomboys'. Even today, very few husbands look after their children full time, with the wife assuming the role of sole family breadwinner.

Only humans with a penis are allowed — as yet — to be ordained priests in the Roman Catholic Church. The social implications of gender within orthodox Islamic states are well known. And politically, the alienation of women within Northern Ireland politics is well documented. For instance, it's not many years since members of the Women's Coalition were told by some of their male counterparts to go home and 'breed for Ulster'.

Inside the Penis

But the penis is amazing not only in terms of its social, religious and political consequences. The penis is amazing in the intricacy of its interior design. It contains as many as three internal, inflatable tubes — hollow caverns, if you like — of erectile tissue.

During sexual arousal, these three channels become engorged with blood. This enables the healthy penis to stiffen, become hard, increase in size and stand erect — and that's just for starters. Two of these inflatable tubes, called corpora cavernosa, run the length of the penile shaft, close to the upper surface of the penis. More or less parallel, they extend from the base of the penis, continue along the length of the penile shaft, ending up at the glans penis — that's the highly erogenous, helmet-shaped head of the penis.

The glans penis is exposed when the foreskin is rolled back, or constantly so in the case of a circumcised man. It's important that the foreskin of infants and young boys should not — repeat not — be forcibly peeled back to reveal the glans penis.

The Penis During Sexual Arousal

At the base of the penis, the two parallel corpora cavernosa diverge and are covered with muscle. Each corpus cavernosum is attached to the lower part of the hip bone or pelvis.

The corpora cavernosa's muscular grip of the pelvis enables the fully engorged penis to stand erect. It is the mooring or hook for the thrusting erect penis during intercourse. The muscles surrounding the corpora cavernosa at the pelvis also help to expel sperm at ejaculation.

Each corpus cavernosum has an artery running through its centre. Each artery has a complex mass of side-shoots. These deliver blood deep into the erectile tissue, enabling the penis to swell in length and width during sexual arousal.

With sexual stimulation, blood rushes into these side-shoots. Where once a tiny tributary ran, now blood rages and surges like a roaring torrent. What were minutes before minuscule pockets of blood become radically transformed into full and swelling lakes. The once flaccid penis stands ready and, usually, willing for sexual activity.

But that's not all. A third inflatable tube — the corpus spongiosum — runs along the underside of the penis. This is thinner than the corpora cavernosa but it, too, enables the once flaccid penis to become bigger and harder. The corpus spongiosum is a continuation of the glans penis. At the base of the penis, this inflatable cavern is attached to a fibrous membrane, further contributing to the stability of the erect penis.

Simultaneous Orgasm

You should be particularly grateful for the little-known bulbospongiosus muscle (or bulbocavernosus) which surrounds the corpus spongiosum at the root of the penis. It's the rhythmic contraction of this muscle — also called the accelerator urinae or the ejaculator urinae — that largely contributes to the pleasure of sexual climax or orgasm.

Women have a similar bulbocavernosus muscle called the sphincter virginae, which covers the bulbus vestibuli — the enclosed entrance at the mouth of the vagina. In heterosexual intercourse, when your bulbospongiosus muscle and her bulbocavernosus muscle dilate at the same time, you have a simultaneous orgasm.

The Urethra (exit route for urine and semen)

The corpus spongiosum contains the urethra — the tube through which urine and semen exit the body. In women, the urethra is only three centimetres long. But a man's urethra is considerably longer, more like 20 centimetres long.

The urethra in men begins at the bladder, runs down the middle of the prostate gland, passes through the tissue connecting the pubic bones, and then extends through the length of the penis inside the corpus spongiosum. Urine from the bladder is finally expelled from the body at the urinary meatus — or the opening — which is normally, but not always (see Hypospadias below), situated in the glans penis.

During sexual arousal, the increased swell of blood in the erect penis blocks the entry of urine into the urethra — leaving the urethra exclusively reserved for the flow, and eventual ejaculation, of semen.

Hypospadias

A hypospadias is a common, penile congenital defect where the urinary meatus is located underneath, rather than at the tip of, the penis. In as many as one in every 200 to 300 males, the urethral opening is on the underside of, or even beneath, the glans penis. In some men, it is found along the length of the penis, in front of the scrotum or even near the anus.

Most cases of an unusually situated urinary meatus are mild and require only minor surgery or even no treatment whatsoever. Severe cases tend to occur in men with poorly developed external genitalia. These men can require major surgery.

Erections

As most adolescents learn — sometimes to their acute embarrassment — erections are involuntary. They occur, beyond the control of the owner, by stimulation of the parasympathetic fibres which cover a man's external genitalia. Parasympathetic fibres cover the prostate and seminal vesicles too.

The parasympathetic nervous system is that part of the body's nervous system which regulates involuntary functions like slowing the heart rate, increasing gland activity and relaxing sphincter muscles.

The involuntary nature of erections is important because men, especially those who have been sexually abused, can become confused by their sexual responses during abuse —

they can feel vulnerable to accusations that they 'enjoyed' it. If survivors of sexual abuse knew about the parasympathetic system, they might more readily place the blame for sexual abuse squarely where it belongs — with the abuser (see also Chapter 18).

Most men have erections — again involuntarily — while asleep. They can occur perhaps as often as five times a night, each lasting for periods of up to 30 minutes. Likewise, women have clitoral erections during sleep.

Even babies and toddlers have erections. So, too, can men who have been castrated, that is, who have had one or both testicles removed.

Size

The size of the penis varies depending on age, temperature, arousal and honesty. When flaccid, adult penile size mostly ranges from 3 to 6 inches. The good news for males on the shorter end of this scale is that the smaller organ tends to extend by a proportionately greater extent during sexual arousal. And, stallions with an extra-long organ can make intercourse uncomfortable for some women, due to excessive pressure on the ovaries.

The average size of the erect penis measures 6.3 inches along the upper surface from the base to the tip of the glans. The most common range is between 5.6 and 7 inches long.

Penile Problems and Diseases

Like any bodily organ, the penis can develop problems or become diseased. Knowing what to look out for, and what you should do if problems arise, could help to reduce discomfort or pain, prevent impotence, stave off — yes — penile amputation, and forestall an untimely death.

Problems with the Foreskin

The foreskin of the uncircumcised male keeps the glans penis moist and highly sensitive to touch. The glans penis of circumcised males — men whose foreskin has been removed for health, religious or cultural reasons — tends to be tougher and less sensitive to touch. But if the foreskin renders the uncircumcised male more sensitive to sexual pleasure, it can cause problems too.

The foreskin is stuck to the glans penis at birth and gradually separates. Sometime between 4 and 17 years of age, full retraction of the foreskin becomes possible, that is, the foreskin can be pulled back to fully uncover the 'helmet' of the glans penis.

It's important to note that this slow process of disengagement must not be hurried along. If you're concerned about the slow pace of this process, consult your physician. But do not force the foreskin to fully retract before the time is right. To do so could tear the tissue and cause a phimosis.

Phimosis

A phimosis is a tightness at the opening of the foreskin. It can develop, at any age, at the site of a foreskin tear. Men with a tight phimosis can have trouble urinating. The foreskin might swell up and retain urine, which can leak out later on. Men with a phimosis might experience pain during masturbation or sexual intercourse. They will usually need to be circumcised — which can be a painful procedure in adult men.

Smegma

The foreskin should be gently retracted to the extent that it has disengaged from the glans penis and washed each day. Care should be taken not to tear any remaining adhesions.

Failure to wash the glans penis every day can result in the formation of smegma — a foul-smelling mix of bacteria, yeasts and urine. Poor personal hygiene could also leave males more susceptible to developing cancer of the penis in later life.

It's important to gently replace the foreskin to its original position after washing. Failure to do so can result in a paraphimosis.

Paraphimosis

This is a painful and serious condition that can be caused by the failure to ease the foreskin back to its original position. The glans penis, in effect, can be strangled by the rolled-back foreskin — which acts like a tourniquet to prevent blood reaching the glans penis.

Men who develop a paraphimosis should see a doctor immediately. If they ignore it, gangrene of the penis can result. If in doubt, get to a doctor immediately. Urologists tend to advise most men who have had a paraphimosis to be circumcised.

A paraphimosis can be caused by the failure on the part of a doctor to return the foreskin to its normal position after a medical examination or procedure — such as when a catheter has been inserted through the urinary meatus to drain the bladder. But it's usually due to the man's own failure to ease back the foreskin after washing or sex.

Balanitis

This is a common inflammation of the glans penis, which becomes red and itchy. Males of every age can get it. It can be caused by poor personal hygiene, as an allergic reaction to soap or by unprotected sex with a woman who has vaginal thrush.

It is usually treated with an anti-fungal cream. Whether one or both partners have it, unprotected sex should be avoided until both partners are in the clear. Failure to do so can result in the partners continually reinfecting each other. If contracted as an allergic reaction to soap, avoid scented soaps, use water-based creams or wash the glans penis only with water. If balanitis persists and is very severe, circumcision can sometimes be required.

A related condition is balanitis xerotica obliterans. With this condition, the area around the urethral meatus (the opening in the penis through which urine and semen leave a man's body) becomes white, while the glans penis and foreskin harden and scar. It can lead to a narrowing of the water passage and the affected man can have difficulty urinating. Sometimes caused by a failure to wash beneath the foreskin on a daily basis, the condition mainly affects older men — but boys can also get it.

Antibacterial and antiinflammatory creams can be applied to the penis to treat it, or it may require circumcision. An accompanying procedure to widen the urethra (the tube through which urine and semen flow through the penis) can sometimes be performed at the same time.

Peyronie's Disease

Men suffering from Peyronie's disease have an abnormal curvature of the erect penis. Erections can be painful and the condition can make intercourse difficult, painful or impossible.

It's caused by changes in the corpora cavernosa whereby soft, erectile tissue is replaced by harder plaques. During an erection, the penis curves towards these hardened, less elastic plaques. Surgery may be required to remove them. Alternatively, the surgeon could compensate for the plaques by removing soft tissue from the other side of the penis.

Priapism

This is a condition where a man is left with a prolonged and often painful erection, unsolicited by sexual desire. It is associated with blood disorders like leukaemia and sickle cell disease. It can also result from the incorrect use of penile injections used to counter impotence. It can sometimes occur after masturbation or sexual intercourse.

The corpora cavernosa swell up, causing the erection, while the glans penis and underside of the penis may remain flaccid. No time should be wasted in getting to a doctor — failure to do so could result in complications, including impotence.

Leukoplakia

This is a rare condition in older men where large white patches appear on an inflamed glans penis. Although painless, it can be pre-malignant and it must be treated in order to prevent the development of cancer.

Cancer of the Penis

This is also rare. Like balanitis, it has been linked to poor personal hygiene. Elderly men who notice a raised ulcer, or discharge, under the foreskin should have it checked out immediately. Treatment may require radiotherapy or, if the cancer is advanced, radical surgery, which may involve the amputation of part or all of the penis.

CHAPTER 2

The Testicles

The testicles — also called the male gonads, the testes (two testes; one testis) or, simply, the balls — are sometimes seen as encapsulating the quintessence of manhood. Not having balls is synonymous with being a coward; having them implies bravery, guts or the reckless pursuit of a goal beyond considerations of personal safety.

The testicles symbolise power, potency and energy. Sperm, manufactured here, can father offspring and is the gateway to future generations. Testosterone is also formed here — the quintessential male hormone.

Women have testosterone too (formed in the adrenal gland, above each kidney). But even in women, testosterone is the male, or androgenic hormone. Testosterone stimulates growth and weight gain, which explains why some sports cheats use it. It also causes acne, in men and women. Men who feel depressed by the state of their skin might be a bit consoled to know that they have an abundance of the male hormone.

The testicles are formed inside the body but, by birth, they have usually descended to the scrotum. However, one in every hundred boys — and as many as one in ten premature males — are born with at least one undescended testicle. Both testicles will be undescended in a quarter of these cases.

When boys are born with undescended testicles, the testes tend to descend naturally before the boy's first birthday. But it's important to confirm that both testicles have descended by the end of the first year because men with undescended testicles have a higher likelihood of developing testicular cancer. If either testis hasn't dropped to the scrotum after 12 months, surgical intervention might be required.

An undescended testicle cannot produce sperm because of the higher temperature inside the body than in the scrotum. That's one reason why the scrotum exists — to provide a cooler environment outside the trunk of the body in which sperm can be produced and flourish.

Millions of sperm are produced inside each testicle, in tubes called seminiferous tubules, while testosterone is secreted in the space between these seminiferous tubules. After its formation, sperm flows to the head of the epididymis — a natural lump that can be felt on each testicle.

The Epididymis and Semen

The epididymis is a tightly compacted duct or tube which measures an impressive 6 metres, or 18 feet long. The tail of the epididymis leads to the vas deferens, which stores sperm and pumps it from the epididymis during ejaculation.

Every man should learn to recognise the feel of the epididymis on each testicle so he can distinguish it from any other lump he might discover while conducting a testicular self-examination (see below). Urologists recommend that men carry out a testicular self-examination about once a month in order to detect any unusual lumps. By knowing the feel of the epididymis, a man won't panic when he feels it — and he'll be quick to spot something that shouldn't be there.

Having been manufactured in the scrotum, semen travels via the vas deferens upwards and back inside the body. It mingles with a sugary fluid flowing from each of two seminal vesicles situated above the prostate gland. This sugary fluid provides energy for the sperm, a packed lunch as it were, to help it complete its journey forth to fertilise a woman's ovum.

Semen also contains prostaglandins which are potent, hormone-like fatty acids which have the capacity to coax the neck of the womb — the cervix — to open slightly. This enables sperm to pass through the cervix and, possibly thereafter, to fertilise an ovum.

Testicular Problems and Diseases

As with any bodily organ, problems or diseases can develop in the testicles. All too many men ignore testicular problems and, whether through ignorance, embarrassment or a gormless macho mind-set, some delay consulting a doctor until pain becomes unbearable; by which stage irreparable damage can sometimes have taken place. So, if you have, or ever develop, any of the following, get to a doctor without delay.

Torsion of the Testis

This condition happens when the spermatic cord twists around itself. It's a very painful and serious condition. But don't writhe on your bed and hope it will go away. It won't. Get to a hospital immediately.

The affected testicle will swell up, feel very sensitive and parts of the scrotum can change colour. It usually affects the left, rather than the right, testicle.

The twisted cord will prevent blood reaching the testicle and epididymis. Partial interruption of the blood supply can cause atrophy of the testicle — a wasting or shrinkage in testicular size. If the twist completely cuts off the blood supply, the affected testicle can become gangrenous within six hours. But the testicle can usually be saved if surgery is carried out within four or five hours.

Torsion of the testis can occur at any age but it more commonly affects infants in their first year and younger adolescents. Some males are congenitally predisposed to it. It can also occur following trauma or injury to the scrotum such as after a kick or a painful, close encounter with the handlebars of a bicycle.

Hydrocoele or Hydrocele

This is a painless build-up of fluid along the spermatic cord or in the membrane surrounding the testicle and epididymis. It can be caused by: an injury; a blockage in the spermatic cord; inflammation of the testicle or epididymis; or, occasionally, a testicular tumour.

A congenital, recurring hydrocoele can occur where the gateway through which the testicle descended into the scrotum — in the womb or early infancy — remains open. Surgery can be required to prevent this happening again.

A doctor will often decide to leave a small hydrocoele alone, but a large hydrocoele is usually drained with a syringe under local anaesthetic.

Epididymal Cyst

This is another kind of swelling in the scrotum. We have seen that the epididymis is the normal lump on each testicle. But a small epididymal cyst — or a number of cysts — can develop on one or both testicles, especially in men over 40. They contain a clear liquid and are harmless.

But men should consult a doctor to make sure they are epididymal cysts and not testicular cancer. Epididymal cysts can be removed if they increase in size, but they are usually left alone.

Spermatocoele or Spermatocele

This is another usually painless swelling in the scrotum. Like the epididymal cyst, it is harmless — but the spermatocoele contains semen. A spermatocoele is indistinguishable from an epididymal cyst unless it is drained and the contents examined. As with epididymal cysts, a doctor will usually ignore a spermatocoele unless its size causes discomfort; in which case it can be surgically removed.

Testicular Cancer

This is the commonest form of cancer in young men aged 15 to 44. It is among the top four killers of young men. Every man has a one in 273 chance of developing it. If caught in time, it can be cured in 95 per cent of cases — which explains why early detection is so important.

Many urologists recommend monthly testicular self-examination to check for unexplained lumps. But not everybody agrees that this is a good thing. Some argue there is no evidence that this leads to earlier diagnosis of testicular cancer. They believe that such a strategy fills hospitals and clinics with the 'worried well' — perfectly healthy men who have just dis-covered the epididymis. But that's not an argument against self-examination. Rather, it is evidence of the need for better education, so men can tell their epididymis from their elbow — and thereby know if a lump presents cause for concern.

There are true stories of men of various ages who failed to consult a doctor until a testicle had swollen to the size of a grapefruit. With testicular cancer, delays make treatment more complex, costly and less likely to succeed.

Testicular Self-examination

The best time to examine the testicles is when the scrotum is warm. So do it when you're having a bath or shower. Use your two hands. Very gently roll or glide one testicle between the thumbs and fingertips. Feel it glide between your fingers. It should feel soft and smooth throughout — apart from the epididymis. Take care not to twist the spermatic cord which could cause torsion of the testis.

You may notice that one testicle is larger than the other — that's normal. If you feel a swelling, don't panic. It doesn't mean you have testicular cancer. It could be a harmless hydrocoele, a spermatocoele or simply varicose veins around the testicle. But you should have it checked out without delay, just to be sure.

CHAPTER 3

The Prostate

Men are more likely to know the location of a woman's cervix than their own prostate. This is odd because the vast majority of men will encounter prostate difficulties in the course of their lives, while more than a third of them will need prostate surgery.

Men have a 50 per cent chance of developing benign prostatic hyperplasia (BPH), an enlargement of the prostate which obstructs the flow of urine from the bladder. Some 14 per cent of men in their 40s have symptoms of BPH, 24 per cent of men in their 50s, and 40 per cent of men in their 60s.

Although so many men have symptoms of BPH and some are driven demented by it, few men talk about it seriously — even to good friends. A man who needs to keep excusing himself from his circle of friends to visit the loo is more likely to be the butt of jokes than to be supported by them in what can be a depressing and wearing condition.

'The waterworks' can act up in any or all of the following ways. You could have difficulty starting the flow of urine; experience an interrupted flow; notice a weaker flow than previously; have a sense that the bladder hasn't completely emptied; experience dribbling after you've left the loo; have increased urgency (having to dash to the toilet in a hurry); or increased frequency (having to urinate more often than before).

These symptoms, especially increased urgency and frequency, can seriously lessen your quality of life. You may

need to constantly interrupt your sleep — and your partner's —
to use the loo; have to stop visiting the theatre; or be forced to
abandon a recreation of choice.

What is the Prostate?

The prostate is a chestnut-sized gland located between the
penis and the bladder. Its function is to make the fluid of the
semen in which the sperm swim. Women do not have a prostate.

The prostate encircles part of the urethra, that is, the tube
urine passes through from the bladder to the penis. As men
grow older, the prostate grows bigger. This can constrict the
flow of urine, like a weight compressed against a hose-pipe.

The prostate can be felt from about two to three inches
inside the anus. That is why a doctor, needing to examine the
prostate, performs a digital rectal examination. Wearing surgical
gloves, he or she will feel the prostate by inserting a finger into
the anus.

If the thought of a digital rectal examination stops you
visiting the doctor to have the prostate checked out, don't let
it. It can be an essential, simple and painless procedure to establish if the prostate needs further investigation.

Benign Prostatic Hyperplasia (BPH)

'You've no idea what it's like to live with him,' says the wife of
a 68-year-old chronic BPH sufferer. Her husband has hardly
returned to bed when he needs to get up again to go back to the
toilet. Nowadays, they sleep in separate rooms.

A 54-year-old man explains that if he has lunch and goes to
the cinema he 'can't last throughout the movie'. Atypically, he
has suffered from symptoms since he was in his 20s. He needs
to go to the toilet three or four times before going to bed: 'If
I'm lucky I get two and a half hours sleep. I've had this since 22
years of age.' He says it's no way to try to impress a woman —
needing to get out of bed five times a night or having to explain

why he carries a two-litre milk container in his briefcase. He takes a critical view of the claims of surgeons and pharmaceutical companies: 'There are people who have gone under the knife or use medication who still suffer.'

Another man in his late 60s began to have symptoms of BPH five years ago: 'Sometimes you're piddling all night. Then sometimes you can't go. You want to but can't. Or you think you're finished, go back to bed and you're up again in five minutes. Yeah, I've mentioned it to my friends — good friends, but never in detail.'

A 61-year old talks about how, if and when it does come up among friends, it would be only as a laugh and a joke. 'But nobody's prepared to say it's a problem for them. Men are very secretive. They keep themselves to themselves and do nothing about it. They never talk about their own problems — they talk about their wife's problems or joke about "the old prostate on the go again".Why doesn't he talk seriously about it himself? You'd feel you'd be setting yourself up for the butt of a joke. They're always talking about their nose, eye or some old sports injury but not about the prostate.'

Men with BPH or waterworks problems should visit their general practitioner. Don't leave it until the symptoms get worse, and don't assume that nothing can be done about it. By ignoring it, treatment could later prove less effective. Moreover, the doctor will want to check if the problem is BPH or, perhaps, prostate cancer.

Your GP will probably ask you to fill in a World Health Organisation score-card which provides objective criteria for gauging the severity of your symptoms. This checklist asks you to rank on a scale of 1 (not at all) to 5 (almost always) answers to a series of questions.

Questions include whether you felt in the past 30 days that you hadn't completely emptied the bladder after urinating; if you felt the need to urinate within two hours after last using the toilet; if you stopped and started several times while urinating; if you experienced urgency; if the flow was weak; if you had to strain to begin to urinate; or if you had to interrupt your sleep to use the toilet.

As well as the digital rectal examination and asking you to fill in the prostate symptoms score-card, the doctor or specialist may also carry out blood tests, urine tests, ultrasound scans or a urine-flow test (where you urinate into a special toilet which measures the rate of flow).

There are several options for treatment. The first is 'watchful waiting', that is, leaving well enough alone. This is often the best strategy if symptoms are not too disruptive of a man's quality of life — and so long as the presence of prostate cancer has been ruled out.

A second option for men with more severe symptoms involves the use of drugs like alpha-blockers or hormone inhibitors. Alpha-blockers relax the prostate's grip on the bladder, while hormone inhibitors inhibit the enzyme that breaks down testosterone, causing waterworks problems.

If you're unlucky enough to suffer a complete blockage, catheterisation may be required. A tube is inserted into the penis under local anaesthetic and the blocked urine flows out through it.

The third option for treating BPH is surgery. For some, this can be the best course of action. Various procedures are available, including stents and TURP (see below).

Stents

These are expandable implants put into the urethra in a minor operation. They are relatively easy and quick to implant. They prevent the prostate from narrowing and so prevent a blockage of the flow of urine.

TURP

Transurethral prostatectomy or TURP is a procedure whereby a surgical instrument is inserted through the penis, under general anaesthetic. With the help of a fibre-optic light, the surgeon removes tissue from the constricted part of the prostate.

TURP can result in retrograde ejaculation, that is, the sperm is catapulted to the bladder rather than through the penis at ejaculation. If this happens following a TURP, the chances of fathering a child are greatly reduced. It shouldn't affect a man's ability to have an erection but, for psychological reasons, some men may experience reduced libido afterwards.

TURP can sometimes result in dribbling problems but these don't always last and can themselves be treated. About one in five men who have had a TURP will need a second one within about eight years.

Prostatitis

This is an inflammation of the prostate gland, often due to an infection. Symptoms can include heightened urgency and frequency, or a burning sensation during urination. Aches or pains in the genitalia, rectum or lower back, or any pain experienced during ejaculation, are also associated with prostatitis. It is usually treated with an extended course of antibiotics.

Prostate Cancer

More men die with, rather than by, prostate cancer. But the number of men with prostate cancer is staggering: up to 30 per cent of men in their 50s and up to 70 per cent of men in their 70s have prostate cancer. Many of them, probably quite happily, don't know they have it.

But a lot do know: three times as many men die from prostate cancer as the number of women who die of cervical cancer — yet there's relatively little awareness of it in the general population. It is the second most common cause of death by cancer in men.

Early identification of prostate cancer improves the chances of successful treatment. However, men often don't know they have it until the cancer is quite advanced. This is because symptoms of prostate cancer usually don't manifest themselves in the early stages. It is also why, increasingly, middle-aged men are being urged to have an annual digital rectal examination.

As we have seen, BPH constricts the flow of urine through the prostate because the blockage develops along the urethra — the tube through which urine flows from the bladder. So the man with BPH knows something is wrong when the waterworks act up.

But prostate cancer usually starts on the outer side of the prostate gland. The man might feel no pain and there may be no perceivable change in the waterworks. In fact, prostate cancer is often discovered during a digital rectal examination when a man presents with BPH. It can also be identified through simple blood tests.

Other symptoms of prostate cancer include: difficulty passing urine, urgency to urinate, a sense of not completely emptying the bladder, blood in the urine, weight-loss or lower back-pain. But, as we've seen, several of these symptoms are similar to BPH — so having these symptoms does not necessarily mean that you have prostate cancer.

Prostate cancer tends to develop very slowly and the doctor might recommend that no action be taken other than to monitor its development. Remember, more men die with it than by it.

Prostate cancer can be successfully treated with female hormones. Possible side effects of these can be diminished libido, impotence or breast enlargement.

Radiotherapy is another option. This is applied to the location of the tumour. A further option, in some cases, is to surgically remove the prostate, the tumour or the testicles.

PART II

Men's Hearts

CHAPTER 4

Men and Heart Disease

Heart disease kills more men in the Western World than any other disease. It accounts for more than a third of all deaths of men aged between 45 and 65. In Ireland and the UK, nearly half of all men die from heart disease and related conditions like stroke.

In Ireland alone, heart disease 'wipes out the size of a small town every year,' says Professor Ian Graham, a consultant cardiologist in Dublin. 'Every man is immortal until it happens to them' but men have trouble personalising it, he says. That's until they get wheeled into the coronary unit of a hospital. There, the old teachers' maxim 'one see is worth a thousand tells' is proved true. Regrettably, many don't live to learn the lesson; and of those who do, it's a pity it takes a heart attack before they cop themselves on.

A Man's Heart

Your life depends on the beat of an organ that you cannot see. A man's heart is about 5 inches long, 3 inches wide and 2.5 inches thick — about the size of your clenched fist. It weighs between 280 and 340 grammes and pumps blood throughout your body at the rate of about 70 beats a minute — that's some 2.5 billion heartbeats in 70 years.

Men at Risk

The main risk factors for heart disease are: being male; smoking; a family history of heart disease; high blood pressure; high cholesterol; being overstressed; eating a diet high in saturated fats; being over 40 years of age; having uncontrolled diabetes; being overweight; and leading a sedentary lifestyle.

A male non-smoker in his 30s with normal blood pressure and cholesterol levels has less than a five per cent risk of a heart attack in the next ten years. But a male smoker of the same age with raised blood pressure and raised cholesterol has up to a 20 per cent chance of a heart attack over the same period.

A 40-year-old male smoker with raised blood pressure and cholesterol has up to a 40 per cent chance of a heart attack in the next 10 years. His non-smoking male friend of the same age with normal blood pressure and cholesterol has a risk of only between 5 and 10 per cent.

Symptoms

The symptoms of a heart attack can include: sudden and severe chest pain, which can extend to either arm; difficulty breathing; sudden sweating; nausea or vomiting; or urgency to perform a bowel motion.

But you won't necessarily experience all of these symptoms if you're having a heart attack. Older men who are having a heart attack might simply feel suddenly tired and breathless.

What to Do During a Heart Attack

If you are, or think you may be, having a heart attack, complete rest is essential. Don't dismiss it as bad indigestion or a cramp across the chest. You should always act as if it is a heart attack. If it isn't, you will do no harm. But if it is, and you dismiss it as something else, it could kill you. The first two hours after a heart attack are critical.

Stop all activity. Do not contemplate walking or driving to the hospital. Get someone to call the emergency services by dialling 999 or 112, making sure they ask for a cardiac ambulance. In rural areas, where the ambulance may take some time, the nearest doctor should also be called. He or she may be needed to stabilise you, or to resuscitate you if your heart stops.

While lying on your side, loosen — or have someone else loosen — your clothing at the neck, chest and waist. And don't panic. If you panic, you will release adrenaline into your system which could compound any damage to your heart.

Prevention

Dr Ciaran O'Boyle, professor of psychology at the Royal College of Surgeons, says that behaviours cause heart disease. Men see health as 'important but not urgent'. They know the heart and blood vessels need activity, but nevertheless 'many men sit on their butts all day'.

Exercise

To take care of your heart, you should exercise most days of the week for about 30 minutes a session, such as by taking a bracing walk with the dog. But check with your doctor before starting any new fitness routine, especially if you have had heart trouble before.

It is often a matter of literally taking a step to a healthier heart. For instance, use the stairs rather than the lift, get off the bus a stop or two early and make sure you get out to stretch your legs during your lunch break.

Food and Red Wine

Eat at least four portions of fruit and vegetables a day. Cut down on fat and fries, reduce your salt intake and lose excess weight (see Chapter 5).

There's evidence that a glass of red wine a day is actually good for your heart, because it is thought to reduce blood-clotting. But drink alcohol in moderation. For men, that's 21

units — not pints — per week. One measure of spirits equals
1.5 units while a pint contains two units. The quota shouldn't
be saved up for a weekend binge but should be spread evenly
over the week, with some alcohol-free days.

Smoking

Don't take your next cigarette — the journey of a thousand
miles begins with a single step. Count the cigarettes you don't
smoke. Record them. Tick them off and reward yourself generously for your achievement. Calculate the money you have saved
on a daily basis and buy yourself something you'd really like with
the money saved. If, or when, you relapse, don't crucify yourself with guilt. Bask in the achievement of the number of
cigarettes you didn't have. And don't take your next cigarette . . .

Blood Pressure and Cholesterol

Check out your blood pressure (see Chapter 6) and cholesterol
level (Chapter 5) from time to time. High blood pressure and
cholesterol are associated with an increased risk of having a
heart attack or stroke.

Breaking with Unhealthy Family Lifestyles

Although family history is a factor in heart disease, it isn't
necessarily caused by congenital defects. Sometimes adult children replicate unhealthy lifestyle behaviours practised in their
family of origin, such as lack of exercise, high salt intake, a high
fat diet, smoking or over-consumption of alcohol.

Stress

Reduce unhealthy stress-levels if you want to live life to the full
(see Chapter 7). If something has to give in your work, make
sure it's not you. One self-employed man learned after his heart
attack to politely tell his bank manager to back off. He reduced
his sales targets and set himself a much healthier objective — to
take a long walk every day.

CHAPTER 5

Men: Food, Fat and Flab

Men in Ireland and the United Kingdom have the highest rate of premature death caused by heart disease in the European Union. A high-fat diet is understood to play a significant role in this carnage. Yet relatively few men approach flab-loss intelligently or take the necessary long-term view.

Fat Versus Sugar

Firstly, it is fat, rather than sugar, which makes you fat. It's the fat — not the sugar — in biscuits, cakes and tarts that piles on the weight. If you want to reduce weight, cut down on fat, rather than sugar.

That's because sugar increases the body metabolism. When you eat more sugar, your metabolism increases too, to burn it off. But fat cannot be burnt off any quicker. If you eat fat faster than you can burn it off, you get fat. So if you are overweight, eliminate the butter, rather than the jam, from your bread.

However, this is emphatically not to encourage you to eat more sugar, which is very bad for your teeth (see Chapter 22). Sugary foods should only be eaten sparingly, infrequently and never to excess. The point is that the primary cause of weight-gain is not sugar — but fat.

Long-haul Weight-loss

It's important to take an intelligent, long-term view if you want to lose weight for good. Short-term crash diets are bad for you:

you will quickly put back on whatever weight you hastily lost.

If you take the long-term view, you can make specific choices that lie within your control which will lead to lasting weight-loss — and you will become attentive to unhealthy habits which contributed to your becoming overweight in the first place.

The person who loses weight speedily might scoff at the less dramatic weight-loss of the man who takes the long-term view. But the man who is in it for the long haul is acquiring sustainable habits, whereas the impatient man learns nothing new. Sooner or later, he will relapse into unhealthy eating habits, because crash diets are unsustainable — his excess weight will come back with a vengeance.

But if you make simple choices, such as cutting the fat off meat, the skin off chicken and substitute fruit for confectionery at break-times, you will lose an impressive amount of weight over a period of two to six months. The smart game is to substitute a healthy action for an unhealthy habit.

You do not have direct control over your weight. But you can control whether or not you eat that biscuit or choose a banana instead. If you concentrate on the small, specific decisions that face you in the here and now, and choose intelligently, your weight will look after itself. So stop measuring your weight and, instead, enjoy the challenge of the next decision that confronts you.

Weight-loss — which will come — will be gradual but certain. And you will become increasingly in command of what you eat. Let your body work out the payoff in its own good time.

Osteoporosis in Men

Adult men do not need any saturated fats. You should cut out full-fat dairy products from your diet and opt for low-fat varieties. But men do need to guard against osteoporosis, the bone-wasting disease that is often wrongly assumed only to affect women. Men can guard against osteoporosis by consuming at least a pint of low-fat or skimmed milk every day, or by taking other low-fat dairy products and green leafy vegetables.

Good Fat and Bad Fat

Men need to eat fat — but only good fats. Good fats (mono-unsaturated and polyunsaturated fats) oil your system. But bad fats (saturated fats) clog it up — leaving you susceptible to a heart attack or stroke.

You don't need a doctorate to know which fats are good or bad for you — although you'd be forgiven for thinking you did. A good rule of thumb is: the fats you get from biscuits, cakes, sponges, gâteaux, puddings, full-fat dairy products, ice cream, cream soups, cream sauces, pâté, peanut butter, egg yolk and red meat contain bad fat (saturated fat), which is in turn converted into 'bad' cholesterol.

Two custard creams contain as much fat as one mini-butter, while a sausage roll contains the equivalent fat of three mini-butters. Would you swallow a spoon of fat at your 11 or 4 o'clock break? You wouldn't? So avoid that biscuit and grab some fruit instead.

You get good fats from oily fish, olive oil and oils like rape-seed, wheat germ and sunflower seed. Olive oil is the best source of monounsaturated fat, which lowers 'bad' cholesterol (LDL-cholesterol). But even good oils should be used sparingly.

Men with Anorexia and Bulimia Nervosa

While eating disorders like anorexia nervosa and bulimia nervosa occur more frequently in women, it is wrong to assume that men do not suffer from them too. Anorexia nervosa can and does affect adolescent males and young men, with one male suffering from the condition for every nine females who do so. Anorexia is a disorder where the person tries to lose weight by induced vomiting, abuse of laxatives, excessive exercising or voluntary starvation.

Males suffering from anorexia can become impotent or, if the condition begins before puberty, it can delay the process of puberty. It can also cause low blood pressure, constipation, vulnerability to infections and serious problems with vital organs like the heart, brain and kidneys.

Men also suffer from bulimia nervosa. It affects one man for every nine women who have the disorder. The man binges on food and then deliberately vomits to avoid weight-gain. He may also abuse laxatives and starve himself. The condition can affect the heart and kidneys, and damage the teeth.

Males with anorexia and bulimia nervosa should discuss the eating disorder with their GP. They could also benefit — as could most people — from good counselling or psychotherapy. There is no shame in being male and suffering from these conditions, so do get help (see Useful Addresses).

Some Tips for Healthier Eating

◆ Full-fat mayonnaise, and foods containing it, pile on the pounds. Avoid it, or choose low-fat varieties.

◆ Add a little spice to your life. Spices, herbs and garlic are a great substitute for salt.

◆ Reduce your consumption of red meat to twice a week.

◆ Eat oily fish like mackerel, sardines, herrings, salmon or trout three times a week.

◆ Have a poached egg with grilled sausages and bacon rather than a fry.

◆ Bake or boil potatoes rather than roasting or frying. Choose boiled rice, not fried rice.

◆ Avoid fish cooked in greasy batter, and other foods cooked in a deep fat frier.

◆ Eat lots of brown rice, wholegrain breads, cereals, pasta and beans.

CHAPTER 6

Men and Blood Pressure

If you're the kind of man who can't remember the PIN number of your bank account, a chapter on blood pressure readings and rates might be about as enticing as settling down to read the telephone directory.

But forget your PIN number and a bank official will ask you a heap of questions to establish your identity. Ignore your blood pressure and the coroner could be asking the questions.

Blood pressure kills silently. You get no warning. There's no flashing light or reminder in the post that you've overspent your overdraft limit. You simply don't know you've got it — even though you could be courting disaster. Then, out of the blue, you could get a heart attack or have a stroke.

This is why high blood pressure, also called hypertension, is known as the silent killer. The only way to outwit this serial killer is to find out if he is prowling around inside your body, ready to strike. You seize the initiative by having your blood pressure regularly checked. The information that that check provides could save your life.

Blood pressure surges when your heart pumps. Then, it dips between beats. That's why blood pressure values are given as two numbers. The first number — the higher one — gives the rate during a heartbeat. The second, lower figure reveals the blood pressure between beats.

A healthy young man in his 20s might have a high or systolic pressure of 120 and a low or diastolic reading of 70. The same guy at 50, if he stays in good shape, could have a high value of 150 and a low reading of 80 or 85. But if he hasn't managed his health successfully, or if he has been unlucky, his systolic blood pressure could be 180 or 200, and his diastolic count 100. Systolic values over 160 and diastolic readings over 95 are regarded as high blood pressure.

Blood pressure varies considerably at different times of the day. It is lowest in the middle of the night when you're asleep, and it usually peaks four or five hours after you wake up. If you have high blood pressure and you're in the throes of a traffic jam or prone to losing your cool at a board meeting at noon, take it easy.

Blood pressure works like this: your heart pumps, then relaxes, repeatedly. While the heart relaxes, blood still needs to get to your brain. So while your heart is taking its well-deserved short break between beats, your main arteries take over. The main arteries contract when the heart rests, making sure blood continues to flow to and through your brain. If the main arteries failed to pump blood to the brain, you would have a blackout and become unconscious.

If fat is clogging up your main arteries, the arteries become narrower and they can't pump blood properly to the brain. When not enough blood gets to your brain, your diastolic blood pressure falls.

To counteract this, your heart has to pump harder to get enough blood to the brain — because your brain simply can't work properly with an interrupted blood supply. Your heart goes into overdrive to ensure a continued blood supply to the brain.

But to do this, your heart has to cut short its well-deserved rhythmic snooze between beats. It doesn't like missing its nap. That's overtime — all the time — doing work the inefficient main arteries should be doing.

Hearts, like people, need a rest. A rest-deprived heart won't go the distance. Men with clogged-up arteries can wear out their heart or have a heart attack. Moreover, the brain wasn't built to persistently receive blood from the heart at that heightened blood pressure — so the danger of having a stroke is also increased.

How to Reduce High Blood Pressure

Blowing your top, sex and physical exercise get your heart to pump faster, increasing your blood pressure. Sex and physical exercise are usually good for your heart. But blowing your top, losing your cool or 'seeing red' — as the blood literally rushes to your brain — is not good for you.

Relax

Blood pressure spikes during anger (Chapter 8) — an emotion men seem to manifest more frequently than women. Some men need to learn how to deal with the stressors in their lives, especially if they're verging towards the volcanic (see Chapter 7).

It can be infuriating when the builder hasn't turned up for the umpteenth time despite promising, yet again, that he would do so. The recognition that life can be unfair is a lesson often not accepted by men. But instead of cursing the slings and arrows of outrageous fortune and forever feeling obliged to put things right, men need to learn to accept the things that cannot be changed.

Garlic

If you do blow your top and suspect your blood pressure is rocketing towards Mars, you could do worse than stuff your face with garlic. Studies have shown that three cloves of garlic can significantly reduce blood pressure in an emergency — but if you do have heart failure, don't take it personally if nobody wants to give you mouth-to-mouth resuscitation.

Salt

Salt is associated with high blood pressure. Reduce salt intake, in the cooking and on the table. If you must have salt, use a little in the cooking rather than on the table.

Avoid salted nuts and crisps. Go easy on rashers and bacon. Choose fresh meat, fish, soups, vegetables and other foods rather than tinned, packaged or smoked varieties. In the main, if it had to be preserved, there could be a lot of salt in it. Check out sauces and gravies for salt content. There's generally a huge range of healthy fresh foods available. Lap them up.

Kill the Weed, Cut Down the Booze

Smoking (see Chapter 4) and excessive consumption of alcohol are associated with high blood pressure. Men shouldn't exceed 21 units a week (see Chapter 5). Red wine taken in moderation could be good for your heart and actually reduce blood pressure. The humble glass of water can be good for the blood pressure by preventing dehydration.

Don't Take your Next Biscuit

Reduce your saturated fat intake and any excessive weight (see Chapter 5). Carrying extra body weight forces your heart to work harder than is good for you.

Check Out your Fingerprints

Your fingerprints can indicate whether high blood pressure is due to your lifestyle or if it could also, or even solely, be due to a genetic condition over which you have no control. Men with a single whorl fingerprint tend to have higher blood pressure than men without any fingerprint whorls. The more whorls you have, the more likely you are to have high blood pressure.

Medication

Lifestyle changes can be at least as important as medication, but your doctor might also prescribe anti-hypertension drugs if your blood pressure remains stubbornly high.

CHAPTER 7

Men and Stress

Check out your jaw. If you're holding it tighter than you need to, chances are that you're over-stressed. And if stress is manifesting itself through a clenched jaw, a tensed-up stomach or an inability to sleep well, what might it be doing to your heart?

For some men, being over-stressed is virtually a status symbol — way up there with the size of their wallet, car or wiggly bits. It's as if being stressed proves they've a big part in the play of life. They're movers and shakers, wheelers and dealers, throwing shapes in the world and strutting their stuff. But being over-stressed is associated with heart disease. That's hardly surprising because any experience of stress has an immediate impact on the body.

In ape-man days, we fought the tiger or ran like hell. Hormones were unleashed, heart rates soared, blood sugar increased, breathing deepened, oxygen shot to muscles, circulation was re-routed and testicles hit base. Man stood primed for action. Today when nasty bills and tax demands roar through the letter-box the very same physiological reaction transforms us, but neither fight nor flight are on any more and our coiled bodily springs stay taut.

According to psychologist and psychotherapist Brendan Madden, stress manifests itself differently in men and women. 'Stress is an emotionally upsetting experience but men tend to feel more constrained in expressing their emotions. Men in work situations often express their emotional unease through aggressive behaviour.

'Women may have a network of support in female colleagues in whom they can confide and with whom they feel freer to express their emotions. Many men may regard the expression of emotion as a sign of weakness and internalise their negative feelings of anger, frustration or fear.'

So, in fact, the man who scorns his female colleague for showing her emotions in a stressful situation may actually be coping less well than she is — and setting himself up for stress-related problems such as a heart condition down the line into the bargain.

'Men need some stress to respond to challenges in sport or at work. When they achieve their goal that kind of stress is not detrimental,' says Madden. Indeed, some stress is needed to get up in the mornings. Any worthwhile, realistic goal we've set ourselves will increase our stress levels. So too will it expand our consciousness, implant self-esteem and help us become more human — and better men. 'However, if a person feels under pressure in a relationship or if his skills are not up to challenges in his job, he suffers unproductive stress which is very detrimental.'

According to Madden, the physiological responses are different for those who don't achieve their goals: 'Cortisone and other corticosteroids are released which suppress the immune system when you're under continuous stress but don't achieve your goal.' Studies have shown that over-stressed individuals will soon get sick — if they're not sick already. Not only are they more prone to heart attacks and strokes, they'd win wooden spoon trophies for catching colds and flu.

Excessive stress impairs your thinking. It diminishes creativity and clamps your brain — may even tow it away. 'Men under pressure to perform may be less creative in their job and their thinking can often be more rigid,' says Madden. 'They can become more indecisive and find it harder to make logical decisions.'

Employers and managers are increasingly recognising excessive stress in the workplace as an obstacle to productivity and profitability. Fionnuala O'Loughlin, a psychiatrist at the Bon Secours Hospital in Dublin says: 'Some companies are beginning to wake up to it. Stress affects performance. It ranges from being under-worked to overworked or having responsibility without power to implement change.'

Work has become more stressful with performance targets, contract employment, information overload, constant change and a new emphasis on individual accountability. But, like debt, stress won't go away by ignoring it. It builds up, advancing steadily towards our personal stress thresholds. Every stress we experience leaves us more vulnerable to the next beast of prey which stalks our path.

Men ignore at their peril the classic symptoms of stress: palpitations of the heart, a knotted stomach, a dry mouth, overeating or loss of appetite, headaches, muscular aches or rapid breathing, hitting the booze, sweating, working too hard or doing nothing at all, panic attacks, absentmindedness, a sense of lacking control over one's environment, a feeling of helplessness and insecurity, diminishment of sex drive, incapacity to perform sexually or brewing anger into depression.

So what's a man to do? Elizabeth Lawlor, clinical psychologist at the Dublin County Stress Clinic in St John of God Hospital, Stillorgan, recommends 'self-observation' — head-to-toe body scans to identify areas of tension. Through its cognitive behavioural stress management programme the clinic educates people in self-awareness, self-care and healthy coping strategies such as exercise and relaxation.

It's plainly silly to suggest that stressful situations don't exist: incontrovertibly they do. And it is sometimes necessary to change the stressful situation or avoid it. However, strictly speaking, situations aren't in themselves stressful — it is you who react with stress to situations. You might love dogs but find speaking in public traumatic — your twin brother might captivate an audience with a great spiel but seize up at the sight of a poodle. Often, you can't change a situation, but you do have the power to change your reaction to it.

Admitting you've a problem with stress is the crucial turning point. Wake up to your body and learn to listen to it. Learn calming, breathing exercises, join a yoga class, relax in a sauna, have a massage or go for a walk. Eat healthily, sleep well and take time out.

Finally, take perfectionism by the scruff of the neck and consign it to a pit with an unfriendly Rottweiler. Decide when you're going to stop work, do the best you can in the designated time — and then knock off.

By the way, how's your jaw?

PART III

Men from the Inside Out

CHAPTER 8

Men and Anger

Men tend to find it easier to get in touch with anger than any other emotion. The man who wouldn't admit to feeling jealous or afraid will possibly readily admit to — and manifest — feelings of resentment, anger or rage.

Once felt, anger can overwhelm a man. The angry man can seem to embody anger itself — with clenched teeth, glaring eyes, taut muscles and tightened fists. The challenge for men is to have the anger, rather than letting it have them.

Some adult men, many of them in positions of power and influence, have never learned a basic lesson in self-knowledge, namely, that other people do not and cannot 'make them angry'. Anger is not — and cannot be — caused by other people. True, another person's words, actions or omissions can trigger my anger. But they do not cause it. The words, actions or omissions to which I reacted with anger could lead to quite a different response in someone else.

This is neither pedantry nor a semantic game. It is a key point for men who have difficulties with controlling their anger. Accepting responsibility for one's own anger — rather than blaming someone else for it — can enable men for whom anger is a difficulty to gain control over their rage. My anger is mine and mine alone. And I am responsible for what I do with it and for the consequences of how I deal with it.

While anger is neither good nor bad, good or bad consequences can of course result from how I deal with it. The problem for some men is that once anger is aroused, it can quite literally disable their common sense. A person acting out of anger has temporarily lost — or perhaps never saw — the wider picture. Whatever he does will probably make matters worse.

Psychotherapist Brendan Madden describes anger as a toxic emotion which can have a negative impact on health, stress levels and relationships: 'We have little or no control when we are swept by anger. However, we do have a say in how long it will last and how we choose to express it.'

Anger is triggered by being physically endangered or by attacks to a man's self-esteem. Neuro-chemicals (catecholamines) such as epinephrine are released, which generate a 'rush of anger that washes over us like a wave', lasting at least a few minutes. Simultaneously, there's an adrenaline rush, heightening arousal of the nervous system.

An illusion of power and invulnerability is generated by these high levels of excitation, which can lead to anger being physically expressed. Men seized by anger, with their disabled common sense, can strike out irrespective of the consequences. Anger is fuelled by an 'internal self-righteous inner monologue. The key to diffusing anger in its early stages is to undermine the inner monologue fuelling it,' says Madden.

Reframing the situation in a different light can enable a conflict situation to be seen from another perspective. For instance, if your daughter disobeys you, see the good in it. In other situations in life, she will more readily stand up for herself.

But reframing is not effective at high levels of anger or rage. 'The best strategy here is to walk away and wait for the mental, physical or emotional arousal to subside,' says Madden. However, walking away won't work if we use that time to brood over what has upset us: 'It's important to distract ourselves as well as getting away. Do something pleasant, something that breaks the brooding.'

Assertiveness for Men

Any mindless ape can be aggressive — but assertiveness demands intelligence and social skills.

- It's important to pick the right time to discuss a grievance. Believe in the good will of the other person and, if possible, start off on a positive note.
- Speak in a clear, calm voice, keep good eye contact and stand your ground — not in an aggressive way but with that sense of your right to be there.
- Be specific about the words, action or omission to which you reacted with anger. The other person cannot be expected to deal with: 'You're always lazy and leave me to do everything.' But they're more likely to be able to deal with: 'When you left the dishes at lunch, I felt annoyed because it wasn't my turn to do them.' And being specific means not dragging up stuff from the past. Deal with the present problem.
- You must be genuinely open and listen to the other person's viewpoint, trusting in their good faith. If you don't continue to believe in the good will of the other person, you won't solve the problem.
- As is well known but seldom practised, conflicts are best and most intelligently solved when there's a win-win outcome.

Men, Anger and the Workplace

Resolving workplace anger isn't always as straightforward as using basic assertiveness skills — which isn't to suggest that assertiveness is ever easy. But attempts must be made to resolve anger in the workplace because so much of men's lives are spent at work that workplace anger can have a corrosive effect on men's health.

Psychotherapist Rob Weatherill believes that: 'Once we join an organisation, we automatically regress at a certain level to the paranoid-schizoid position.' That is, we believe 'John is for me' and 'Mary is against me' (that's the schizoid part), and that 'Other people are out to get me' (the paranoid bit). He says the paranoid-schizoid state is a 'readiness to hate or resentment that's applicable to nearly anybody in the workplace'.

Workplaces often hold the myth that we're all getting on and there are no hierarchies. 'But the hatreds and rivalries are still there. People feel deprived of recognition for the work they do. So they resort to stealing, either literally, or by taking sick days. It leads to scheming or plotting against authority — which represents the parent.'

He sees anger in the workplace as more or less universal: 'Even the most intelligent and aware people are just as affected. This makes it difficult for organisations to function. After the initial period of co-operation, people regress back. Managers feel resentful too. They're being attacked, so it is hard for them to be generous. People don't trust more than one or two people in the workplace.'

CHAPTER 9

Men and Fear

What do you fear? Blindness? Losing your job or a big contract? Aspects of your sexuality? Not being able to initiate and sustain an intimate relationship? Making a decision that turns out to be detrimental to you or others?

You could fear being intimidated or bullied by someone at work, by a neighbour-from-hell or even by a member of your own family. You could fear having to speak in public, having to pass a house with a wicked dog or failing an exam. You could even fear success itself and be fearful of how you might cope with success having achieved a goal.

You could suffer separation anxiety at the thought of loved ones dying in a car crash. You could fear casting off a role to which you have become accustomed. Or you could fear declining sexual capacities.

You could fear losing your mind through sickness, a dodgy memory or a descent into insanity. Or you could fear being crushed by depression to the point of despair. Some men have an unarticulated fear of ending their days poverty stricken and on the street, bereft of family, friends and all that was once dear to them.

Men can fear the impulses or desires that are deep within them, which they glimpse in disturbing dreams or wild fantasies. Or they can fear the loneliest and only certain journey of them all, which every man must surely take and take alone — and pray that, in that hour, they will not judge their life to have been lived in vain.

Fears can dictate a man's life. But for all their fears, men tend to be slow to admit to them — even to themselves. They tend to live under the shadow of the myth that fear is not for men. The lad who sensibly declines to put his life at the mercy of the dodgy-looking branch of a tree or chooses not to walk through a busy railway tunnel can be taunted as gutless by his peers — rather than responsible.

That social expectation on males not to show fear is learned early in boyhood. It doesn't let up in adulthood. A man, quite rightly tearful at the death of a loved one, can be told to pull himself together and be strong for others.

Fearlessness seems to pay in a man's world. Evander Holyfield didn't fear the intimidating heavyweight boxer Mike Tyson and he succeeded in pounding that convicted rapist to a crushing defeat. In the subsequent fight, the once-mighty Tyson was reduced to ear-biting before the victorious and fearless Holyfield.

I have witnessed a young farmer stand his ground, arms erect, directly in the path of a stampeding herd of cattle. The farmer did not flinch. Despite their power to crush and kill him, his display of fearlessness prevailed: the rampaging animals applied their leggy brakes — just like in the cartoons. They skidded to a stop in abject surrender, inches from his feet.

It is the fascination of controlling their own fear which draws some rock-climbers to put their life in their own hands, literally. But climbers have to come down from the cliff-face if their fear is too great on certain days.

Culturally, perhaps even genetically, men protect women and children. If somebody really must go downstairs in the dead of night to check out if there's a burglar on the prowl, it's no bad thing that it should be the man. But it's this social expectation, the role of the protector, which tends to bewitch people into believing that real men know no fear — and that they shouldn't admit to it when they do.

Dr Joseph Fernandez, consultant psychiatrist at St Brendan's Hospital in Dublin, feels that what men fear most of all is other people discovering their real fears and vulnerabilities. 'Men fear others discovering about themselves. We're all actors and we don't like to be discovered.'

Fernandez believes that some men structure their entire lives so their fears don't protrude in public performance. They're seen to perform adequately but it's another story in the privacy of their own homes. Men's lives can be blighted by fear and doubly blighted through their failure to admit their fears, even to themselves.

According to Dómhnall Casey, a psychologist and psycho-therapist in private practice in Dublin, men can fear not being in control. They tend to be wilful rather than willing. 'We fear not being boundaried and create boundaries that aren't there. Men find letting go to the mystery of living very difficult.'

He says men can fear their own unconscious. They can fear their sexual and violent impulses because they're not at ease with that aspect of themselves: 'Self-control without insight can be painful. We can't all know what's lurking in the deep. We don't all confront our deeper demons. Each of us has a different demon. Obsessionals fear losing control; psychopathics fear being vulnerable; hystericals fear being abandoned.'

Men can also fear their emotions. They can be afraid of letting go of pain, of crying their own tears. Casey says some of his male clients come in full of bravado and strength. Within minutes, they might be crying and say, 'I don't know where that came from.' Other men won't let go of anger or grief sensing that if they cried they would cry a river. Casey believes that all fear has a spiritual root. 'Part of the male fear is the dissolution of the ego. That takes place on a spiritual path. We're all headed for death and most men are afraid of it.'

CHAPTER 10

Men and Jealousy

It's not easy for a man to tell his partner he feels jealous. The vibe at the prospect of telling her — especially if he hasn't done it before — is decidedly uncool. He can feel it will demolish his masculine street-cred and give her too much power over him. After all, he's still got his pride. Coming out from the mask of invulnerability to admit to jealousy can seem too costly a risk.

Check it out in the courts. Time and time again you hear of assaults on women, children and other men motivated by jealousy. This unspoken emotion often leads to assault, battery and violent murder.

Jealousy is a universal human experience, yet men don't often talk about it. They'll sing about it (Tom Jones's 'Delilah': 'I felt the knife in my hands and she laughed no more'; John Lennon's 'Jealous Guy'; Led Zeppelin's 'Heartbreaker'; Joe Jackson's 'Is She Really Going Out With Him?') but when's the last time you heard a group of guys in the pub talking about how they manage feelings of jealousy?

Jealousy can flood men with an intense sense of inadequacy and an abject fear of abandonment. It can carry with it delusions of infidelity and catapult a man into states of panic and terror. He sees the woman as emotionally more powerful than him. Feeling unequal and threatened, he doubts his lover's commitment to the relationship.

Some psychologists believe it all goes back to a boy's closeness with his mother and the painful realisation in time that it's

Daddy she's married to, not him. Watch any toddler muscling in and breaking up his parents' hug. The plot is sown deep within us in real life before we've even heard our first fictional story of the eternal triangle.

Clive Garland, a psychotherapist specialising in men's issues at the Clanwilliam Institute in Dublin, says that if men feel insecure in their relationship they can feel jealous. When they're jealous — and he believes it's a normal phenomenon — Garland says that the best thing men can do is to tell their partner how they feel: 'Most men try to play it cool and not admit they're jealous. Find a way to talk it out with your partner. If you can go over to her and tell her you're feeling jealous and insecure, you're on a winner.'

Garland believes that men who fail to manage their jealousy become possessive and feel the need to control the other person. The need to control is a way of avoiding feelings of jealousy.

'Men's jealousy has far more implications for women's health than for men's health,' says Róisín McDermott, chairwoman of Women's Aid. 'Jealousy can lead to paranoia in the man. He believes he owns her.' McDermott disputes the explanation, or even sometimes the justification, for murders of women as crimes of passion: the if-I-can't-have-you-nobody-will concept. 'She's dead. He's alive. Why didn't he kill himself if it was a crime of passion?' she says, urging men to recognise that jealousy is self-originating rather than caused by a woman's behaviour.

Psychotherapist Rob Weatherill says that jealousy is a universal social sentiment which is not revealed very often because it's not seen as appropriate. He associates it with the child's inordinate demand for love and recognition. Men who were damaged or repeatedly humiliated as children will be more likely to be in need of recognition and more likely to control their partners.

Alluding to Freud, Weatherill says that jealousy can involve an unacknowledged homosexual love for the rival male.

Primordial energies and passions and the denial of the homosexual element are very strong: 'The two men are more likely to kill one another for their (repressed) love for one another — not for the woman. The woman is incidental.'

Rob Weatherill believes the jealous man's repressed homosexuality has the potential to attach to any other man, real or in fantasy.

Dr Harry Ferguson, senior lecturer in the Department of Applied Social Studies at University College Cork, says jealousy is hugely denied but pervasive. He sees it as part of the masculine shadow. Violent men convince themselves their partner is having an affair. This forms part of their rationale for battering them. For the jealous man 'other men are perceived as threats to the integrity of the man's estate which is jealously guarded'.

Left unchecked, normal jealousy can become a pathological condition called morbid jealousy. Dr Art O'Connor, consultant forensic psychiatrist at the Central Mental Hospital in Dublin, says that jealousy can become all consuming and dominate a relationship. The morbidly jealous man can accuse his partner of having affairs. He searches the woman, checks her underclothes or looks for semen on the sheets. Combined with alcohol, morbidly jealous men are dangerous and can kill, although Dr O'Connor has also seen homicide cases where the morbidly jealous murderer is a dry alcoholic.

For most couples, all that is required is for men to say 'I feel jealous' or, for less brave souls, 'I'm feeling a bit left out.' More often than not, this self-disclosure will lead to reassurance and a healthier relationship than before.

CHAPTER 11

Men Coping with Loss

M en seem to be at a disadvantage, and often appear not to cope well, when they encounter loss in their lives; while women tend to be emotionally better equipped, and to receive greater support, in dealing with critical losses.

A man whose child has died is more likely to be asked how his wife is, than how he himself is coping with his bereavement. When a marriage ends through death, separation or divorce, men tend to be less able to face the world alone than women. Generally, widows cope better, and live longer, than widowers; while separated or divorced women tend to fare better than their male counterparts.

Separation and Divorce

Separated and divorced men who do not live with their children can ache every day living apart from them, as was so eloquently expressed by Bob Geldof when he said: 'I can feel my insides being turned inside out. Without my children I'm nothing.'

The experience of the separated father cut off from his children was powerfully explored by Robin Williams in the film *Mrs Doubtfire*, based on Anne Fine's insightful novel, *Madame Doubtfire*.

Men can face an uphill battle in trying to win custody of their children. The growing realisation that the law affords fathers so few rights is an injustice increasingly highlighted by men like Bob Geldof, in his attempts to win custody of his children, and by John Waters, in his pioneering articles on the subject in *The Irish Times*.

Separated fathers who want to do so are encouraged to establish and remain in contact with their children soon after separation or divorce. Fathers should avail of family mediation services (see Useful Addresses) rather than enter a bruising legal battle. They should continue to develop their parenting skills (Useful Addresses) and never break an appointment with their children.

Families Need Fathers, a UK organisation providing advice to separated and divorced parents (see Useful Addresses), recommends that fathers avoid agreeing to a period of no contact with their children. They warn against an undefended divorce, saying that undefended allegations can limit a father's contact with his children. And they advise careful consideration before leaving the family home, lest the father be not let back in, even to see his own children.

Deserted Husbands

Deserted husbands do not receive the same degree of financial support from state welfare provision as deserted wives receive, despite all the talk of equality. And deserted husbands tend not to receive the emotional and social support in their parenting that mothers can more readily receive from networks like mother and toddler groups.

Men and Miscarriage

People are becoming more aware of the impact a miscarriage can have on a woman, and rightly so. But a man can also be deeply affected by his partner's miscarriage or the stillbirth of a child. While the mother is naturally more intimately involved — after all the new life was within her body — the man too can be profoundly affected by the loss.

Studies at the Coombe Women's Hospital, in Dublin, have shown high stress levels among the male partners of women who have had a miscarriage. The research, published in the *Journal of Obstetrics and Gynaecology* in 1996, showed that although supports were provided for the women, a substantial majority of men, whose son or daughter had been miscarried, could not find any emotional support for themselves at the time, despite manifesting high states of psychological distress.

Redundancy and Retirement

Men often seem to go downhill soon after retirement, while a man whose job is made redundant can feel as if his entire self-esteem has been swept aside. Men can all too easily think and feel that they themselves have been made redundant, whereas, in fact, it is the job which has been made redundant.

Given that men readily identify with their job, they can feel as if they themselves have been discontinued, discarded, placed on the scrap-heap or deemed surplus to requirements.

The removal of their predominant role in the family, which is still so often that of breadwinner, can strip men of their dignity and pride. Their self-esteem and confidence can plummet, and many men can go on to experience impotence, depression, alcoholism, and some, in despair, take their own life.

Men Dealing with Loss

Confronted with a critical loss, it can be difficult for some men to get in touch with how they really feel. It is all too easy to bury their feelings, 'put it behind them' and try to get on with their lives.

Men tend to protect themselves with rationalisations, platitudes and a deft change of subject. They're feeling fine and coping grand thanks very much and how are you keeping yourself? It's as if some men need to give themselves permission — or to be given permission — to let themselves feel how they truly feel deep down. It can be harder for them to name and claim an authentic, self-originating feeling, take time to sit with it, and let tears, if needs be, well up from within. Tears, for men, are so often seen as a weakness instead of the strength and poultice for grief which they can so readily be.

Men can have difficulty finding the words to express uncomfortable emotions. Some men are like foreigners learning a new language. It can be hard enough for them to feel the emotions swirling around inside, without having to find the words to express them too.

Men need to enter bravely into, and not seek to deny or suppress, the feelings of shock, anger, guilt, confusion, depression and whatever other emotions accompany the experience of a significant loss in their lives.

Men's sense of themselves, how they defined themselves, their role in society, the status they felt they had acquired and which they projected on to others' perceptions of themselves, can be torn asunder by a critical loss.

Men experiencing loss can feel humiliated, insecure, a failure and deeply hurt. But these feelings can be seen as, and become, an opportunity to grow and establish a new sense of self. This is not to suggest that this is ever easy. It isn't. Nor that men would willingly trade what they have lost for this new understanding of themselves. They wouldn't. But once a critical event happens, however harrowing it may be, it can lead to new hope and a new understanding of the self not based on a job, an income or a relationship — which, by their nature, have to pass away.

If a loss is felt deeply, faced intelligently and lived well, a new sense of self can emerge, with a more firmly based self-identity and well-grounded self-esteem not dependent on other people or transitory things.

Socrates summed up his entire philosophy with the simple words: 'Know thyself.' The experience of loss, no matter how painful, can be an opportunity, even an invitation, for men to do precisely that.

CHAPTER 12

Men Coping with Depression

It feels like you're stuck underneath a scrum. But you don't know when it'll get off you. You're feeling suffocated and freaked out. Just powerless,' says a 25-year-old male construction worker who suffers from depression.

Despite being handsome, healthy and attractive to women, he admits to 'very low self-esteem', although he knows intellectually there's no reason for it. He fears his employer might see him as a liability if he knew about his depression, but despite this he has told his foreman and a workmate in confidence.

When he is well, he's an excellent worker — efficient, responsible, hard working. But when he's depressed his motivation implodes. He can't relax or even think straight. He gets anxiety attacks. And he misreads harmless comments as personal attacks and takes them to heart. As he puts it: 'Someone says boo to you. You take it the wrong way. It echoes around your head.' When he's depressed, he finds himself 'losing the rag over nothing'. His self-esteem plummets 'like an uncontrollable force telling you you're worthless'.

But most of the time his bouts of depression don't affect his work. In fact, he believes men who suffer from depression can be more responsible than others. As he puts it: 'Just because someone's depressed doesn't mean they're a health hazard. Men who get depressed are more likely to do a good job than those who are carefree. They're that bit more in touch with themselves.'

Work is so important to men that their job can help them to cope with depressive tendencies. It can act as an antidote to depression. Little wonder, then, that unemployed men or retired men can be vulnerable to depression. And men with depressive tendencies can become depressed when they go on holiday.

During vacations, the bulwark of tasks, deadlines and a clearly defined function in society are stripped away. Men's various roles — banker, shop assistant, builder, manager — are temporarily removed. Self-loathing can bubble to the surface and cast a man into despair.

Depression can be triggered by what are objectively insignificant things — like being unable to fix something as simple as a bicycle puncture. A man can go from 'I can't fix this' to 'I'm no good at practical things' to 'My whole life is a cascade of failure.' A man sinking into a depression might have a panic attack, where he's suddenly fretful, his body-temperature might change dramatically or he might weep or sweat profusely. Or he might experience the onset of depression less dramatically but feel helplessly flattened beneath that crushing weight.

Dr Patrick McKeon, consultant psychiatrist at St Patrick's Hospital in Dublin and chairman of Aware, an organisation that helps people with recurrent mood disorders, says men who get depressed tend to be more hardworking and conscientious than others. They so undervalue themselves that they seek, through their excellent work performance, to prove their value. He believes depressive tendencies are virtually a basic requirement for certain jobs. Creativity and depression go hand in hand. 'If you want people who are creative, you can't have one without the other,' he says.

Depression has been described as anger turned inwards. If we are angry with someone but cannot express the anger in a healthy way, the anger can seep inwards, turning into depression. We could be angry that a partner has left us through death or divorce, or that a car driver maimed or killed someone dear to us, or that someone committed a crime against our property, a loved one or ourselves.

Men can also feel angry with themselves. Perhaps a behaviour or omission has caused hurt or injury to the man himself or someone else. Maybe the man realises his misery is self inflicted, that he misjudged a situation, took what turned out to be a wrong path. Men can be forced into a situation where they have to admit to themselves or others that they were selfish, fearful or self-deluded; and, perhaps, that they ignored a more manly, magnanimous or honourable path that lay within their grasp if they had but cared to look.

Depression brewed from anger can be associated with the discovery of the shadow side of our motivation, the recognition of the ignoble part of what drives us. Men can realise that beneath the apparently worthy pursuit of perfection lies a craven need to avoid anger; or see their service to others is driven by a need to be needed; or that a driven pursuit of success is fuelled by a need to avoid failure at all costs.

Insight into what we are angry about can liberate a man from depression, which can sometimes be linked to experiences of childhood abuse. Insight into personal motivation can be painful; but it can open a man up to a world beyond his own manufactured importance and bestow on him an awareness of the world beyond his own needs and obsessions.

Charles Handy observed that a man's family is rarely impressed by what men tend to view as their achievements — career progression, business success, fame or fortune.

A wife or children can seek very different things from their husband or father than the trophies men tend to chase and regard as important. They can look for a quality of presence in the man, a capacity to truly listen or simply the gift of the man's time to play or celebrate with them.

Insight into personal motivation, and a recognition of what a wife or children really want, can liberate men from the tyranny of blind alleys, unsatisfying pursuits and worthless male trophies. The challenge for men can be to enrich the quality of their own relationship with themselves and with those who are dear to them.

Tips for Men who Feel Depressed

◆ Accept depression when it comes. You are not a freak. Many men and women feel depressed and crushed from time to time.

◆ Seek human support and a helping hand. Tell your partner or a good friend how you feel, or ring a depression helpline (see Useful Addresses). Visit your GP, counsellor or therapist for a consultation.

◆ Over 80 per cent of even severe depressions can be successfully and speedily treated by non-habit forming drugs and psychotherapy.

CHAPTER 13

Male Suicide

S uicide is a major cause of death among males aged 15 to 24 in Ireland. The male suicide rate more than doubled between 1976 and 1994, reaching some 18 per 100,000 towards the end of the period. And the rate of male suicide rose even further in the late 1990s.

Although depression (Chapter 12) is twice as high in women, 4.5 times as many men as women take their own lives. Three times more Irish males between the ages of 15 and 24 are taking their own lives than 25 years ago, and researchers insist that this is not merely a reflection of improved reporting of suicide. Four times as many young men kill themselves in Ireland as in 1990 and this is 'not in any way related to more accurate reporting — it's a real increase,' says Dr Patrick McKeon, chairman of Aware, an Irish association which helps people with mood disorders.

Some 3,000 people lost their lives in more than 25 years of the Troubles in Northern Ireland, but four times that number took their own lives in Ireland during the same period. Most of them were men. While virtually the same number of women attempted suicide, men succeeded much more often. If women's suicide attempts can be interpreted as a cry for help, the male success rate suggests men feel they are beyond help — or they lack the personal and social skills to ask for it.

International studies show that young unemployed men up to 25 years of age are especially vulnerable to suicide. They seem to feel bewildered and confused about their role in society, a bewilderment partly triggered by the increasing presence and effectiveness of women in the workplace.

High alcohol consumption, marital breakdown and isolation from traditional family supports like the extended family are also factors leading to an increased incidence of young male suicides. Moreover, cultural shifts like declining religious observance can set young male psyches adrift, leaving them more susceptible to suicide.

Studies show that most people who take their own lives suffer from some kind of psychological or psychiatric condition, such as depression, mood disorders, schizophrenia or alcoholism; but that is not to say that most people with these conditions try to end their own lives.

However, a recurring characteristic in many who do take their lives is the inability to cope with rejection. The break-up of a relationship, a row with a family member, losing a job, not being picked for a team, social isolation for being gay — any of these can trigger a feeling of rejection and public humiliation. Women suffering rejection tend to seek and get support from a social network and circle of friends. They tell someone how they feel. But some men seem to feel that self-revelation of personal difficulties is tantamount to an admission of failure of their masculinity or manhood. They find no healthy release for pent-up negative feelings and so are more likely to turn to alcohol, drugs or work to escape from their interior pain.

Such men need to learn that needing help — being interdependent — is an integral part of being human. They need to learn that admitting they have a problem does not diminish their masculinity in any way. A telephone call to the Samaritans or a group like Aware, or the experience of honest self-revelation to a friend, can make life worth living — and ending one's life a needless option — and so prevent the torment for relatives that suicide can leave in its trail.

A Father's Grief

I don't understand myself since my son took his life. It's like I feel nothing. I don't have the feelings I feel I should have. It's difficult to feel angry with him. I do feel angry with him but as soon as I feel angry with him I feel guilty, so I stop allowing myself to feel angry. It's like letting myself actually feel how I must be feeling deep down is selfish. I don't want people counselling me. When I suspect friends are getting into counselling mode I switch off. I tell them to back off.

I was never able to talk with him. We never seemed to be able to communicate. One of the last times I saw him, I knocked down a suggestion he made about a new career move. I feel guilty about that. I wonder how differently things might have turned out if I'd listened to his ideas and not knocked them. I just knocked his idea without knowing. Rationally I know that one moment of dismissing an idea didn't make him go out and kill himself. Rationally I know that. But emotionally it's very hard not to feel guilty.

There's a lot of blame about. People in the family are guarded with one another. It's easy to blame, blame myself and blame others or be blamed by others or hear others blame others. We don't talk so much.

The fact is that we'll never know why he did it. We'll never know why. If somebody is knocked down in a road accident you know why they died. It's horrendous but at least you know why. You can be angry with that dead person if it was partly his own fault. But with suicide you just don't know why.

We know of other suicide victims who were all smiles with their family one minute and went out and killed themselves the next. Their parents feel angry that they didn't speak. We saw our son soon before he took his life but he never said what was going on deep down. We don't know why he did it. It's a mystery that nobody will ever be able to answer.

Coping with Male Suicide

The late Dr Michael J. Kelleher, director of the National Suicide Research Foundation in Cork, believed this father spoke eloquently for people bereaved by suicide. Unlike death by an accident, suicide involves a choice. The deceased — more usually a son than a daughter — appears to find his life of no value, and his suicide seems to pass judgment on other people.

All sudden deaths can cause anger. But, with suicide, it is difficult for those left behind to make the 'crucial separation between the act of dying and the person who dies. One feels anger at the fact that he died by suicide,' he said.

The bereaved can feel guilty for feeling angry with the son who took his own life. The work of bereavement in suicide is to make the separation between the manner of death and the person who died.

Dr Kelleher believed that phrases like 'loved one' are best avoided because there is 'no perfect person and therefore no perfect relationship'. With suicide, survivors can reflect back on the relationship and blame themselves. Events and conversations immediately preceding the death can be attributed with an unreasonably high significance.

Dr Kelleher believed that 'emotional matters are independent of time'. The death of a son or husband can lie dormant for years. But people can — and do — come to terms with death by suicide: 'We're fashioned by nature to come to terms with death. People come to terms with the most appalling tragedies.'

CHAPTER 14

Men's Groups

When Robert Bly's international bestseller, *Iron John: A Book About Men*, was published in 1990, it caused a sensation by selling more than a million copies worldwide.

Sociologists and the media were intrigued by its success. Considered the gender and cultural watershed that gave birth to the 'men's movement', it seemed to tap into men's need for a different experience of masculinity. The puzzle was why so many men bought the book, what male needs it met and why its market was so ready to receive it when it did.

According to Edmund Grace, a Jesuit priest, a growing number of men feel the need to meet and reflect on what it means to be a man. He believes there's a support that only men can give to other men and that manhood — contrary to what is often depicted — is a positive value. He says the traditional model for men of the 'tough loner' doesn't work and that both the long-term unemployed and the successful businessman alike can feel hollow, unsatisfied and lost.

He believes a father cannot initiate his own son into manhood, and that it has to be done as part of a wider male community. He speaks of men's 'spirituality' and says: 'We have energies inside ourselves, independent of us. They're positive energies, tied up with being male and human. Reflecting on experiences of being male with other men taps in on those energies and leads to a healthy celebration.'

Kieran McKeown, an economic research consultant, is married for 17 years and has three children. Deeply in love with his wife, he loves his children but feels that there are 'massive expectations around the one adult in our lives'. In his small men's group which meets fortnightly they discuss love, money, children, career, insecurity, power struggles in the workplace and intimate relations with their wife or partner. The group of eight men are all university educated, very articulate and 'fairly middle class'.

He has been involved for several years in men's groups and larger men's gatherings led by people like the US mythologist Michael Meade, an extraordinarily gifted storyteller whose medium is to tell a story, interspersed with a drum beat, to a group of men and invite them to talk about how the story reverberates with them.

McKeown says that it is only in recent years that he would choose to attend a men's gathering. Previously, he feels he wouldn't have been as open or as capable of reflecting on his experience. He says: 'It's a very interactive thing. If you've never done this you'll never see that it's possible to do this with other men.'

Men tend to be their careers — or they're unemployed, he says. 'A more energy-sapping paradigm is hard to imagine. It's the currency men communicate on. I have a career and a business but we're more than just the workforce.'

Ray Smith, a group therapist and community worker, has worked with men's groups over the last 10 years. Usually he works with unemployed men who are concerned to find a job and earn money. Some join men's groups in the hope of getting a job at the end of it; others see the need to change themselves and 'trawl through their own difficulties'; more join to work out a relationship, or because their wife or partner is making demands on them to change.

Dermot Rooney, a clinical psychotherapist and lecturer, says men tend to lack a forum to meet and talk outside work or the pub where the emphasis can be on external things. He attended the first of the men's 'gatherings' in Ireland in the early 1990s at which the eminent Jungian psychotherapist, James Hillman, addressed some 100 men.

Rooney found it profound yet somehow 'frightening' and 'vaguely intimidating'. But it was 'absolutely fascinating'. Using storytelling and poetry, he was stunned by the way men stood up and spoke and he was very taken by the willingness of men to share their insecurities. He sees men as 'trying to grapple with the chaos and yet the mystery of why we're here'.

Rooney stresses there's lots of fun and humour at men's gatherings. Speaking of the men's group he belongs to, he adds: 'There's zero cultishness about it. There's no leader, no structure. The only boundary is that there's no physical violence. There isn't an agenda. The only agenda is for men to talk. It's a quest.'

Catherine Sheehan, who has a masters degree in journalism, recalls a men's conference she attended entitled 'Men and Intimacy' at St Patrick's College in Carlow attended by some 160 people, almost half of whom were women. She found that most men who attended wanted to be better fathers and to break down barriers between themselves and their wives and children.

She was very taken by a talk which got 'thunderous applause' on fathers and sons by Colm O'Connor, a psychologist with postgraduate degrees in applied and clinical psychology. He spoke of men being imprisoned in the patriarchal role and asked what it meant to be a father. Fathers, he suggested, are often known by their absence, by 'shoes on the landing' and the sound of the car driving away in the morning.

Dr Harry Ferguson, senior lecturer in the Department of Applied Social Studies at University College Cork, believes the success of events like the Carlow conference is in large part due to the presence of women. He says: 'A huge amount of learning took place by men and women. There was a powerful and empowering sense of some kind of common ground being worked out.'

He says some men-only events can lead to the demonising of women and a failure to hear women's voices. However, he believes it is legitimate to have men-only events. Single-sex events can challenge men to let go the expectation that women will do the emotional work 'which implicitly challenges men's fear of other men'. He believes men have an agenda to sort out for themselves and they should not depend on women to sort it out for them.

PART IV

Sex and Relationships

CHAPTER 15

Impotence, Libido and Viagra

Men suffering from impotence, impotency or erectile dysfunction are persistently, or periodically, unable to achieve, or maintain, an erection to the point of ejaculation during sexual intercourse.

An occasional failure to achieve orgasm due to factors like fatigue, stress or alcohol (which is well known to increase the desire but decrease the capacity), does not mean you have erectile dysfunction. All that means is you need more sleep, greater relaxation or fewer scoops.

Impotence is sometimes confused with infertility — the inability to father children. Most men suffering from impotence will not be infertile, while infertile men can enjoy fully active and satisfying sexual relationships.

Impotence and erectile dysfunction are usually used inter-changeably. However, technically, erectile dysfunction refers specifically to the inability to have an erection, while impotence is a broader term which includes erectile difficulties and psychological issues like performance anxiety.

Extent of the Problem

The widespread and unexpected demand from its launch in 1998 for the male impotence drug, Viagra (see below), indicates the extent of the problem of erectile dysfunction. It is estimated that some 140 million men worldwide suffer from impotence. Some 40 per cent of men over the age of 40 suffer from it for extended periods. In the US, up to 20 million males attend physicians for the management of impotence, while one clinic alone in Ireland sees up to 60 new cases every week, according to consultant urologist Mr T. E. D. McDermott.

Libido

Most cases of impotence are due to psychological rather than physical causes. A declining libido or reduced sexual desire is often a factor.

Sexual desire can decline some years into a relationship. It can be caused by myriad factors. Sex can become predictable. Children can reduce the opportunities for spontaneous sex. Childbirth can leave your partner feeling sore, and less disposed towards sex, which can break a previous pattern of more frequent sexual relations. Parents of young children can be so sleep deprived that when they get to bed, sex is the last thing on their minds.

Financial and business pressures can reduce a man's energy and interest in sex. Juggling the many and various demands of earning a living, pursuing a career, running a business, paying the rent, keeping healthy and spending some time with your children can leave men with less time and energy for sex than previously.

The possible build-up of unresolved conflict in a relationship doesn't help either. If a man feels niggled or angry with his partner for whatever reason, he could be better employed discussing what's on his mind than wondering whatever happened his libido. Diminished sexual desire can be a warning sign that all is not right in a relationship, and that attention, time and effort needs to be given to it. Or it might simply mean the intensity of the passion in the early years of a relationship has settled down to a less passionate, but perhaps more profoundly loving, manner of being together.

Men experiencing impotence associated with psychological or relationship difficulties could consider agreeing with their partner not to have sex for a designated period. This can take the pressure off the man and dispel performance anxiety. A period of agreed abstinence can give a couple the opportunity to look at issues which might lie behind the bout of impotence. Failure to perform might be just the presenting problem. The things that need to be recognised, discussed and resolved can be very different.

A temporary bout of impotence can be seen as an opportunity to open up to your partner and to grow in trust together. At such a time, impotence can be seen as the calling card or invitation for a couple to explore deeper spiritual issues of acceptance, healing or sustenance in the relationship.

Taking the manly risk of being vulnerable — to open yourself up to the fear of rejection by revealing your inner thoughts or fears — can create the opportunity for a deepened relationship; which, in turn, can revitalise the sexual aspect of the relationship.

During an agreed period of abstinence, as well as talking openly, there is nothing to prevent a couple from touching, kissing or exploring one another's bodies. With the pressure removed to perform sexually, sexual desire, and capacity, can be speedily restored.

A sexual relationship can also peter out if the partners don't take the risk of telling one another what they really like sexually. It's all too easy for a man to assume his partner can read his mind, and then complain that she or he is not satisfying his desires.

By taking the risk of vulnerability, sharing fears and speaking hidden thoughts, a renewed intimacy of minds will often lead naturally and spontaneously to a renewed intermingling of loins.

It can be quite easy to establish if impotence is psychologically based. If a man is impotent with his partner but can sustain an erection to ejaculation by masturbation, or if he has erections while asleep (his partner can confirm this) or upon waking, then the impotence is psychological.

Psychological reasons for impotence can include relationship conflicts or inner conflicts, due to factors such as having been sexually abused in childhood or adulthood.

Men experiencing impotence shouldn't hesitate to seek the assistance of a good psychotherapist. There's no stigma attached to seeking counselling or psychotherapy in order to explore psychosexual issues that could lie behind impotence or diminished libido. A good psychotherapist can enable men to gain remarkable insight into themselves and enable them to make courageous decisions.

Physical Causes of Impotence

Impotence in as many as 40 per cent of cases is caused by physical factors, so it can be important for a man to consult his GP to establish if there is a physical explanation for erectile dysfunction. Below are some of the physical factors that can cause male impotence.

Defective Genitalia

Anatomic impotence is a rare, physical cause of impotence, where the man has defective genitalia from birth or as a consequence of injury to the genitalia.

Surgery

Impotence can sometimes result from surgery to the penis, prostate, bladder or rectum.

Neurological Disorders

Atonic impotence is quite a common kind of impotence brought about by neurological disorders, that is, medical conditions which affect the body's nervous system like diabetes, multiple sclerosis or chronic alcoholism.

Injury to the back or pelvis can also cause impotence by damaging the spinal cord.

Vascular Diseases

Men with poor blood-flow to the periphery of the body can suffer erectile dysfunction. For instance, men with atherosclerosis can have the blood supply to the penis constricted by small, narrowed arteries, caused by plaque formations in the arteries. Alternatively, blood can leak away from valves in the corpora cavernosa or corpus spongiosum (see Chapter 1) in the penis, preventing the penis from becoming, or staying, hard.

Drugs-related Impotence

Certain drugs can cause erectile dysfunction. Antidepressants, and medication for conditions like high blood pressure, angina, glaucoma (pressure in the fluid of the eye) and migraine, can cause temporary impotence.

If drugs you are taking are making you impotent, tell your doctor, who will probably be able to offer an alternative medication.

Lifestyle Factors

Nicotine (smoking), overwork and fatigue, too much alcohol, high cholesterol levels (associated with a high-fat diet), high blood pressure and high stress levels are associated with impotence.

Treatments

Mr McDermott explains that before 1985 the only treatment available was surgical implants (see below). Since then, drugs have become available. The options below provide 'purely physical erections', unaccompanied by arousal. Once a man is confident the erection will work, 'he can concentrate on other aspects of arousal'.

Vacuum Pump

The vacuum pump is a rigid condom-like device. Air is sucked out from around the penis and blood drawn back into it. A rubber ring around the base of the penis maintains the erection. It shouldn't be used for longer than 30 minutes.

The pump is available over the counter at certain pharmacies. You don't need a prescription. Ninety per cent of the cost of about £200 may be redeemable if it's returned within 10 days. The result is 'functional, firm but not as hard as the natural way,' says Mr McDermott.

Surgical Implants

Impotence can also be treated with prostheses — surgical, inflatable penile implants. A hydraulic system is inserted along the length of the penis and connected to a reservoir of fluid and a pump. 'You press a button, up it comes. Press the button, down it goes,' says Mr McDermott.

The penis hardens, but it doesn't get as long or as wide as during a natural erection. Implanting them can involve a three day stay in hospital. They are an option where other forms of treatment fail. Some 80 per cent of men are satisfied with them, says Mr McDermott.

Intracavernosal Injection

This option involves penile injections, some of which your GP can prescribe. They use a vasoactive compound like prostaglandins, a drug which increases the blood supply. Ten minutes later, the penis becomes erect. The correct dose must be used for the erection to last for half an hour. Use too much and you can have a painful erection.

The injection is administered by a syringe, in its simplest form. Although there are other injectable devices, the other forms still use a needle. You could be prescribed this option if you are under stress. Only 25 per cent of men are still using it after a year, by which time they have usually re-established their confidence and they no longer need it. Others don't like it and for others it doesn't work. It gives almost a normal-sized erection.

Viagra

The male impotence drug, Viagra, which *Time* magazine dubbed the 'erection pill', aroused intense media interest from its launch, and a seeming scramble by impotent men — and others — to buy it. In 1998, it became the fastest selling new drug in the US, with some 10,000 prescriptions for it being written every day. Shares in its manufacturer, Pfizer, rocketed with its successful launch.

Viagra is 'the eventual nirvana of them all,' says Mr McDermott, who had it on trial with patients in Ireland and found it to be 'extremely successful'.

In tests, 60 per cent of impotent men said they were pleased with the outcome when they took doses of 25 milligrams, while 80 per cent were pleased when the dose was increased to 100 milligrams.

Side-effects of Viagra

Pfizer acknowledges that possible side-effects of Viagra include headaches (16 per cent), facial flushing (10 per cent), dyspepsia or indigestion (7 per cent), nasal congestion (4 per cent), urinary tract infection (3 per cent), and mild, transient abnormal vision, giving a bluish tinge and an increased sensitivity to light (3 per cent).

There have been reports of men dying having taken the drug but no definitive causal link has been established.

Viagra is not a recreational drug. It is a prescription-only medication to be used solely by men who have been diagnosed by a doctor with impotence or erectile dysfunction.

The doctor's diagnosis is very important, because the physician needs to check the man's cardiovascular condition and health. For instance, you must not use Viagra if you are taking organic nitrates, a medication generally given to people with angina. Of the total male population who have erectile dysfunction, it is estimated that some five per cent will be using organic nitrates.

'Nobody should even think of getting hold of this drug without being examined by a physician,' says a spokesman for Pfizer. It is only for men (and not for women) and only for impotent men. Healthy men will not benefit from taking it but they could experience some of the possible negative side-effects of the drug, he says.

Asked about press reports that Viagra improves the love-making of healthy men, the spokesman said: 'The power of the mind is amazing.' He attributed reported improvements to the placebo effect. That's when an inactive substance can appear to have a positive effect on a condition solely because the person believes it will do so. Any drug trial needs to take stringent account of the placebo effect so as not to distort the findings of drugs research.

An advantage of Viagra is that you don't have to take it routinely. You use it only when you need it. If you are pre-scribed Viagra for impotence, you should not take more than one pill a day and not at all on a sexually inactive day. Beyond that, you will just experience the side-effects with no further beneficial effect.

Experts have warned that overusing Viagra could damage the retina, affecting your eyesight. You should never exceed the prescribed dose. As with any prescribed drug, you should only use the drug in accordance with your doctor's instructions. Generally, it is best taken sometime between 20 minutes and an hour before intercourse. There is a 'window of opportunity' for successful intercourse of between four to six hours after that.

In short, Viagra is not a recreational drug. It should only be taken on prescription, after diagnosis of impotence by a physician. And, finally, it is not an aphrodisiac: in the absence of sexual stimulation, a man, having taken it, will not be aroused.

CHAPTER 16

Infertility and Sperm Count

Male infertility shouldn't be confused with impotence. Impotence is the inability to have or sustain an erection (Chapter 15). Male infertility is the inability of the man's sperm to fertilise the woman's ovum. If a man has had frequent, full vaginal intercourse with a fertile woman for more than a year, without conception, the male partner could be infertile.

Male infertility, which can be temporary or permanent, can be caused by: immature sexual organs; problems in the production of sperm; sperm motility (that is, the ability of sperm to propel itself in semen); erectile difficulties; the failure of the sperm to break through to fertilise the ovum; and certain previous or current medical conditions, or treatments, related to other organs or systems in the body.

It can be due to, or made worse by: torsion of the testes and undescended testicles (see Chapter 2); epididymoorchitis (inflammation of the epididymis and testicle); retrograde ejaculation, as can happen after certain surgical procedures (see Chapter 3); previous gonorrhoea (see Chapter 19); treatments like chemotherapy; and on-going problems like chronic liver or kidney conditions.

An extensive list of certain drugs including anabolic steroids, beta-blockers and even marijuana can also contribute to male infertility. Consult your doctor if you're on medication and you think you are infertile, because there could be a link. But, of course, you must not change or stop taking your medication without the approval of your doctor.

Lifestyle factors have also contributed to male infertility. If you think you are sub-fertile and you're trying to father a child, it could be worth your while drawing up a personal programme which includes some or all of the following:

- Avoid sexual intercourse or masturbation for at least a week before the fertile time in your partner's monthly cycle.
- Don't wear tight-fitting jeans, trousers or underwear; don't soak in a hot bath; don't spend too long in a hot shower; and give that sauna or jacuzzi a miss. All of these behaviours are associated with infertility because they increase the temperature of the testicles. But even normal body temperature is too hot for the manufacture of sperm. That's why the testicles are in the scrotum — it's cooler there than inside the trunk of the body. The activities listed above increase the temperature of the testicles, reducing their capacity to manufacture sperm.
- Stop smoking, drink less alcohol.
- Reduce or eliminate caffeine intake.
- Eat a healthy, balanced diet and lose weight.

Declining Sperm Count?

A vast literature has appeared in recent years examining whether sperm production and semen quality is deteriorating in modern men.

A Finnish study recently published in the *British Medical Journal* said the incidence of normal spermatogenesis, that is, sperm production, decreased in Finnish men from 56.4 per cent in 1981 to only 26.9 per cent in 1991 — that's a deterioration in sperm production by more than half in a mere decade.

Moreover, there was a dramatic increase — from 8 per cent to as much as 20.1 per cent — in the number of men who had complete spermatogenic arrest, that is, they had no mature sperm cells. Meanwhile, men with partial spermatogenic arrest (who had only some mature sperm cells) increased from less than a third (31.4 per cent) to almost half (48.5 per cent).

The study also found that testicles had decreased in weight; they had become increasingly thickened or scarred; and they had smaller seminiferous tubules — the tubes in the lobes of the testicles — than ten years previously.

The study, headed by Dr Jarkko Pajarinen of the University of Helsinki, was based on post-mortem examinations of the testicles of 528 men, who had died between the ages of 35 and 69. Half died in 1981, the remainder in 1991.

Some scientists believe that, while the study suggested that sperm count is deteriorating, it didn't prove it. But there is reason for concern.

Professor Lewis Smith, director of the Institute for Environment and Health at Leicester University, believes the Finnish study was 'not one of the most robust' because its population was not well distributed, nor was there any evidence of their lifestyle. 'However, already ten per cent of the population are sub-fertile. Combined with low sperm count, it is significant. But I would argue the evidence is not yet conclusive. It's alarmist to say we face doomsday but there's enough evidence to take the issue seriously.'

Consultant urologist, Mr T. E. D. McDermott, says the report makes no comment about when the biopsies were taken. 'Logically, when somebody dies the testes arrest because they need blood supply to maintain them. Whether this has an effect on the testes or not is unknown. Certainly the function could be affected by the length of time after death when the testicle was biopsied.'

In what is potentially the greatest challenge to the Finnish study, Mr McDermott says biopsies of a corpse are often un-related to the actual sperm count of the man while he was alive. Recently, he performed a biopsy on a subject whose sperm count was abnormal while alive, yet everything seemed normal in the biopsy.

In 1992, the *British Medical Journal* published a paper by Elizabeth Carlsen *et al.* which reviewed over 60 scientific papers investigating whether semen production had decreased during the past 50 years. It found that the mean sperm count had almost halved from 1940 to 1990 and that semen production had fallen from 3.40 ml to 2.75 ml.

That 1992 report also noted an increase in testicular cancer and 'possibly also' undescended testicles and congenital defects. It concluded that the decline in semen quality was probably caused by environmental factors.

Subsequent reports contradicted these findings, while others corroborated them.

But if sperm production and semen quality are deteriorating, what is causing this decline? The usual suspects are environmental toxins, chemicals, industrial solvents and oestrogen-like substances which mimic female hormones.

Ms Gwynne Lyons, pollution consultant with the Worldwide Fund for Nature, says that higher predators — humans included — are at risk from oestrogen-mimicking substances: 'If you expose rats to these, they decrease their testicle weight and reduce their sperm output.' If seals are fed fish from polluted seas, their pup production can decrease. Otters in the polluted Lower Columbia River in the US have smaller penises and testicles than those from non-polluted areas. All Florida panthers now have undescended testicles. Alligators in Lake Apopka, in Florida, have smaller penises and, increasingly, undescended testicles, she says.

The finger of suspicion is pointing to DDT pesticides, PCBs (industrial chemicals), phthalates used to soften plastics, and bisphenol A, used in polycarbonate plastics and in food tins.

Ms Lyons says: 'More men are being pushed into the infertility region. Epidemiological studies have shown that men in the 1990s have lower sperm count than men in the 1940s. We ignore these warning signals at our peril. We don't have the luxury of being able to wait for proof.'

CHAPTER 17

Sexual Infidelity

Neanderthal man is alive and well and boasting of sexual conquests in a locker room near you. As you put your wet socks on, you have to hear whom he last bedded or is about to lay. He cares less for the objects of his penetration than for his discarded carton of Head & Shoulders; he laughs at victims' love letters, sleeps with other men's wives and he couldn't give a monkey's about the lives and families — not least his own — that he damages.

This is not to scour the indiscretions of the young who plant wild oats in experimental or transitional relationships. Rather, I ask why some men who are happily married or in long-term relationships have an affair or even do a runner. Is there a screw loose in the male psyche that predisposes the likes of Daniel Ducruet to cavort naked with a 24-year-old busty model when he was married to the ostensibly highly desirable Princess Stephanie of Monaco? Or in Bill Clinton who put his US Presidency in jeopardy by his 'inappropriate' relationship with Monica Lewinsky?

'Abandon', I've been alerted, isn't a politically correct word. 'It almost sounds like adultery,' said William Keogh, a relationship counsellor with the Marriage and Relationship Counselling Services in Grafton Street, Dublin. 'People don't talk about adultery now. Nowadays it's an affair. Desert, leave or separate are today's words. And abandon has connotations of men storming out indifferent to consequences.'

A recent *Newsweek* feature had no problem using the A-word. Adultery, it concluded, concerns more the breach of trust than sexual infidelity: 'Today the deepest betrayal is not of the flesh but of the heart.'

Mary O'Conor, a relationship counsellor and sex therapist at the Albany Clinic in Dublin, says it's a bit stereotypical to think of men doing a runner for the sake of a newer model. She is sympathetic to the guys who have affairs. Usually, she says, they have low self-esteem. 'If the person they're involved with is constantly putting them down, withholding affection or sex, if she's constantly criticising him, he won't feel good about himself. Or if the woman wants to change things about the man, it can get too much for him. She wears him down with constant rejection.' Poor spineless lamb, driven by his spouse to infidelity!

Many men get stuck on the chase: for them, the chase is everything. After they get married, they fail to see they're into a whole new ball game. The game is now about managing, rather than achieving, a relationship.

Clive Garland, a psychotherapist at the Clanwilliam Institute in Dublin, believes that many men fear emotional closeness in a relationship. He suggests that these men tend to lack a strong sense of their personal identity, fearing that they'll be smothered by intimacy. They can be tempted to flee the complexity of intimacy by seeking out someone else — 'but you bring the same complexity with you'.

His colleague, Ed McHale, a psychologist and family therapist at the Clanwilliam Institute, says that many men tend to be emotionally illiterate. Not knowing how to be emotionally available to their partners, they can be drawn to fleeting sexual liaisons or protracted relationships of continuous infidelity, returning to the tired old game of chase they've played before. Struck by a new partner's understanding or sexual attraction, they opt for casual or opportunistic sex, free of the burden of having to get involved in a relationship.

Rob Weatherill, a psychotherapist and author of *Cultural Collapse*, believes that men do a runner because they're confused: they no longer know what it means to be a man. 'In the past, men disguised their power over women by becoming their protectors. Women were on pedestals while being considered fair game in exclusively male gatherings. Now with men's political power exposed in the last few decades men are confused.'

Weatherill believes that men react to the feminist critique which mocks the traditional male values of distance, authority, strength and mastery in three ways. They take on board the feminist critique and change their behaviour; they cling to old power and lash out at women; or, in fear of the hidden power of the feminine, they run. 'But it's hard to run because it's an inner problem they're running from.'

Of course, it isn't only men who start affairs. As Ed McHale says, 'The gender with the most power will tend to initiate sex.' As women gain greater power in society, the present imbalance may even itself out.

CHAPTER 18

Male Rape

Every month in Ireland alone, at least one adult male is raped. Most at risk are men in their late teens and 20s but even men in their 40s have been raped. Big, strong men can and have been raped by smaller men armed with knives or syringes. On occasion, victims outnumber but are overpowered by an armed attacker.

Gang rapes of men are also committed. Men are raped by complete strangers, acquaintances, relatives, family friends, lodgers, prison inmates, ministers of religion and even employers.

Women are attuned from an early age to the dangers of rape. The only men likely to be aware of the threat are those who have already suffered it. Men hitching lifts or walking by night generally consider themselves invincible to sexual assault.

If and when men hear of male rape, many tend to react with incredulity. Some disparage the manliness of victims for not having beaten off the attacker — 'I would've punched his lights out' — and presume by twisted logic that the victim must be homosexual.

With crass arrogance and the self-knowledge of an amoeba they are unaware of the vulnerability and abject powerlessness they'd discover within themselves should they ever be raped and be forced to swallow their scorn with every pelvic thrust.

The veneer of the machismo pose was brilliantly exposed as so much hot air in John Boorman's cult film, *Deliverance*, and in Quentin Tarantino's brilliant cinematic achievement, *Pulp*

Fiction. In both, a strong adult male is attacked, a male whose physical and mental strength cannot prevent the rape.

Audiences question neither the manliness nor the sexuality of either character. Yet the message is slow to get through, not only to the tiresome single-celled aquatic protozoan, but even to many male rape victims themselves, that the crime bestows no shame on them — but only on the depraved action of the rapist. It seems many have seen the films but missed the meaning.

'Against your will and by force', sums up the experience of one of the victims in Liam McGrath's gripping documentary, *Male Rape*, televised on RTE, Ireland's national broadcaster. Another rape survivor, a university student, speaks in that documentary of being beaten, raped and urinated upon after hitching a lift from two men after a late-night stint at the campus library. A third explains that he was 'overpowered by him, not by strength but by fear'.

'Men have difficulties presenting as victims of rape,' says Dr Maud McKee of the Sexual Assault Unit at the Rotunda Hospital in Dublin, who believes that the worst effect is an increased confusion about role and gender. 'Apart from the invasion and the trauma, men are uncomfortable with the sense of being overpowered. They feel threatened by that. Control has been removed from them. Some fear people will think they're gay. There are taboos about men coming forward.'

Dr McKee believes that male rape is more an act of violence than a homosexual act. 'It's an abuse of power and a victimisation.' Her views are echoed by Dorothy Morrissey, a counsellor at the Limerick Rape Crisis Centre, who believes that most perpetrators of male rape are most likely to present in their ordinary lives as heterosexuals.

Dr Art O'Connor, forensic psychiatrist at the Central Mental Hospital in Dublin, believes that some homosexual men only express their homosexuality aggressively, perhaps after drinking. Most likely candidates are those who 'in their everyday lives are anti-gay and are trying to cover it up from society'.

Dr O'Connor has also come across cases of young men being raped regularly by someone in authority over them in the workplace. 'The victim is often very afraid for his job. Not everyone has the luxury of being able to move. They can see no way out. It's easy for a stranger to say he'd walk away.'

Olive Braiden, director of the Dublin Rape Crisis Centre, says that even when a young man tells his family, he is sometimes met with incredulity: 'How in the name of goodness could you have let him do that?' According to Braiden, as well as the feelings of shame and degradation experienced by women victims, men also have to handle the questions that arise about their own sexuality. The greater hurt can be to a man's sexual identity.

Eileen Calder, a counsellor at the Belfast Rape Crisis Centre, says that rape emasculates a man. 'What they want is their sense of masculinity back. In some ways men tend to blame themselves more than women. They've the whole issue of whether he should've been able to fight them off.' She adds that some gay men are in relationships that are abusive but they rarely ring the centre to say they were raped by their partner.

Male rape can suggest to the most strident feminist the need to reconstruct her view of men and masculinity: strong men also suffer at the hands of depraved and violent males who would attempt to dehumanise them for their own pleasure. The view that you can't rape a man who doesn't want it is as contemptible and base as the obscenity that women who are raped asked for it.

CHAPTER 19

Sexually Transmitted Diseases

If you think you've caught a sexually transmitted disease (STD) following sexual activity with a partner, it's important to have it dealt with. Go to a doctor or get yourself to a genitourinary clinic. Don't let feelings of embarrassment keep you away. It could, as they say, happen to a bishop. You can use a false name if you feel you must, but don't ignore the condition.

Chlamydia

This is one of the commonest sexually transmitted diseases. It shouldn't be ignored because it can cause conjunctivitis, testicular swelling or even sterility.

Some men have no symptoms but carry the infection and pass it on to sexual partners. Others feel a stinging at the tip of the penis. They may notice a watery discharge and feel pain while urinating. There may be a soiling of underwear or sheets. Symptoms develop up to six weeks after sexual contact with an infected sexual partner.

Treatment is with antibiotics. Diagnosis enables a female carrier to be identified and warned of her condition. If she is not treated, she could become infertile.

It's important for men suffering from Chlamydia not to have sex until their condition has been completely cured.

Genital Herpes

This is a very common STD. Symptoms usually occur up to two weeks after sex with an infected person. The man may have itchy genitals or find it hard to urinate. He might notice swollen glands around the groin or feel feverish. He could have headaches, general aches and pains, darting pains in his legs and generally feel rotten. A couple of days later, a red lump appears on the genitals which turns to a blister and later bursts to form a nasty, weeping ulcer.

Medication is available. Some kinds are for application to the blisters; other medication is taken in tablet form. Medication is most effective if used after the initial tingling warning but before the eruption of the lumps and ulcers.

Safe and limited use of paracetamol can help contain the pain. Make sure the affected area has lots of air. It might also help to bathe the sores with a salt solution several times a day.

Attacks of herpes recur in about 50 per cent of people who have had an initial outbreak. These can be triggered by stress, ill-health, sunbathing, depleted immunity or extremes of temperature. Subsequent outbreaks tend to be less severe than the first occurrence.

Genital Warts

These are lumps of varying sizes and shapes which can be moist and itchy. The warts appear on the penis or anus out of the blue, usually due to sex with an infected person and perhaps years after being exposed to the infection. The doctor can freeze the warts, burn them off with electrocautery, paint them with a cell-killing solution or apply a special acid.

Gonorrhoea

Commonly called 'the clap', gonorrhoea can cause a sore throat, fever and swollen glands in the neck. There may be a yellow discharge from the penis and it can be painful to urinate. Homosexuals are vulnerable to infection of the rectum. Some men will find it is painful to have a bowel motion and there may be a rectal discharge of blood and mucous.

The first indication of a problem tends to emerge within five days of sexual contact with an infected person. Aches or pains can disappear about ten days later but the man should still seek treatment. If he doesn't, he will continue to infect others.

Gonorrhoea is usually treated with antibiotics or penicillin.

Syphilis

A few hours after sex with a person with syphilis, a man's bloodstream is strewn with the infectious bacterium. Up to 90 days later (but it could happen after only a week), a highly infectious, flat, painless, rubbery ulcer forms on the penis, anus or tongue — the site being determined by the nature of the sexual activity engaged in with the infected person. After two months, the ulcer will have healed but a scar will remain. Within two months, the disease can become highly infectious, with some men developing flu-like symptoms, a rash on their hands and feet, swollen glands and oral, genital or anal ulcers.

Syphilis then ceases to be infectious but a third stage will occur within three to 20 years. Body parts like the tongue, nose or bones decompose and the brain itself can begin to be eaten away.

Needless to say, it's important to act at the first stage. Penicillin is usually used. While this can cause a mild reaction, it is as nothing compared with the doomsday scenario of ignoring the condition.

HIV/AIDS

Heterosexual and homosexual males can contract HIV through unprotected sex or by sharing needles, razors or toothbrushes with people who are HIV positive or who have AIDS. Men can also contract HIV or AIDS by receiving contaminated blood through a blood transfusion.

The blood of an infected person must be avoided, a point to be borne in mind during menstruation or if an infected partner has a cut. Condoms should always be used during sex with a person with HIV or AIDS — but bear in mind that condoms can break or come off. Even with condoms, there is an element of risk. Extra strong condoms should be used during anal sex — but a significant degree of risk remains.

Swallowing the semen of a partner with, or who may have, HIV or AIDS is obviously to be avoided. But another risk of engaging in fellatio is that it could be possible to contract HIV or AIDS from the saliva of an infected partner.

Hepatitis B

This is a very serious condition which can be transmitted through heterosexual or homosexual activity, as well as by receiving contaminated blood. Hepatitis B is highly infectious and can cause jaundice, cirrhosis, liver failure or cancer of the liver.

It is widespread. The risk of contracting it by having unprotected sex, especially in parts of Asia, Africa or the Pacific, is very high. You should not share razors, needles or toothbrushes with anyone you suspect could have hepatitis B.

You can be vaccinated against contracting it which, along with a condom, can make sex with carriers less risky. But, even then, a significant risk remains of contracting hepatitis B.

Pubic Lice

These parasites suck blood from the skin around the pubic hair. You can catch them if you have sex with someone who has lice, or even from soiled sheets and towels. Pubic lice are eradicated by using a special shampoo and maintaining a rigorous hygiene routine for towels, underwear and bed clothes.

P A R T V

Man Alive

C H A P T E R 2 0

Men: Shift-work, Sleep and Snoring

Men are more likely than women to do night work and to suffer from resulting sleep-related health problems. Night workers are forty times more prone to accidents, more susceptible to viral infections and suffer poorer physical and mental well-being.

Dr Paul Guèret, a Dublin-based occupational physician, conducted research with Dr Gerry Walpole on the health effects of night work for the Royal College of Physicians of Ireland. Their literature review identified ten nightwork-related conditions.

Men who are Most at Risk from Night Work

Men in any of the following categories should consider requesting a transfer to daytime duties. Under workplace health and safety legislation, your employer may consider it prudent, or in some cases may even be obliged, to accede to your request.

- sleep disturbance: if an occupational physician deems a worker's sleep disturbance to be excessive.
- excessive fatigue: if the work requires high vigilance and an occupational physician recommends a transfer.

- involvement in accidents: workers like lorry drivers prone to dozing off should seriously consider transferring to daytime work.

- gastrointestinal disorders: night workers have a 50 per cent higher chance of developing stomach problems. If the disorder is resistant to normal treatment, transfer to daytime work should be considered.

- ischemic heart disease: Dr Guèret believes night workers probably have a 50 per cent higher risk of ischemic heart disease. Someone who has had a heart attack could consider transferring to daytime work.

- mental illness: Drs Guèret and Walpole recommend that workers with depression (unipolar affective disorders) or manic depression (bipolar disorders) should consider a transfer.

- deterioration of asthma control: some asthmatics are known as 'night time dippers' — they suddenly get worse at night. Their cortisone level lowers so they're more prone to asthma attacks. Asthmatics so affected should consider a transfer.

- deterioration of diabetes control: diabetics are either insulin dependent (they need insulin injections) or non-insulin dependent (they get by with diet control and oral medication). The doctors say it may be in the best interests of insulin-dependent workers to avoid night work. Insulin-dependent diabetics are most at risk where a rotating shift operates.

- deterioration of epilepsy control: sleep deprivation is associated with epilepsy. While epilepsy shouldn't be a bar to doing night work, fits are more common immediately before and just after sleep. Where there's an increased frequency of seizures, a transfer should be considered.

- shift-work maladaption syndrome: most people adapt to night work but some five to 20 per cent of people are permanently intolerant of it. They will suffer from insomnia, have persistent fatigue, regularly use sleeping pills, be irritable, suffer changes in behaviour, perform poorly and develop digestive problems. Men suffering in this way should not do night work.

Men and Shift Schedules

Sleep experts recommend that shift schedules should last for at least three weeks rather than having them rotate more frequently than that. Once a shift schedule has finished, you should have a couple of days off before the next schedule begins. If your schedule is less favourable, you should discuss it with your health and safety representative at work.

You shouldn't feel that, as men, you have to put up with whatever shift schedule is in place. Employers don't want to risk litigation for work-related damage to your health. If they are wise, they will listen to your concerns.

Men and Jetlag

Men who travel a lot can frequently suffer from jetlag. If you're travelling to the other side of the world, perhaps on a business trip, try to travel in a westerly direction. This is especially important if you need to operate at peak performance the following day. Moving west is more in accord with the body's diurnal rhythms and you will suffer less from jetlag. Diurnal rhythms are daily patterns of activity like sleeping and eating — and even regular variations in temperature.

Dr Graham Fry, a lecturer in tropical medicine at Trinity College, Dublin, suggests that when you arrive at your destination 'try not to make any major decisions within the first 24 hours'. He recommends trying to return back home on a Friday, if possible, to give the body time to recover before the following week's work.

The drug, melatonin, can be taken to alter the body's natural diurnal rhythm. You would take a certain number depending on whether you're flying east to west or west to east.

But, as with any drug, there are concerns about its use and it should only be taken with caution, says Dr Fry.

Men and Snoring

Dr Catherine Crowe, a consultant in sleep disorders at the Mater Private Hospital in Dublin, treats a lot of men for snoring. She treats five times as many male as female snorers. Most people are referred to her because they are disturbing their partner's sleep.

Men snore more than women, although women snore too — especially if they are pregnant or after the menopause. But, even then, women usually snore less than men.

Men over 40 tend to snore most of all. While a man snoring will often affect his wife's sleep, women from the late 40s tend to have less continuous sleep anyway — so a snoring man shouldn't take all the blame.

Causes of Snoring

Snoring, whether heroic or more quiet, is caused by the partial or total obstruction of the upper airway. This obstruction vibrates the tissue, generating the noise.

Some snoring is associated with sleep apnoea syndrome, which involves the complete obstruction of the airway at the top of the nose, the palate or at the base of the tongue.

Men with sleep apnoea syndrome can have as many as 400 apnoea a night. Their snoring tends to sound irregular and requires professional attention. They will emit gasps and snorts at the end of each pause.

Technically, these men wake up each time they snore. Although this 'waking' is beneath the level of consciousness, it can be detected on an EEG — a machine which examines the structure of sleep through the application of electrodes to the head of the sleeper.

Men with sleep apnoea don't sleep as soundly as they should and can often feel sleepy during the day. Men with the condition can be unwise to drive because of the danger of falling asleep at the wheel. US studies have found that men with sleep apnoea syndrome are five times more likely to have a road accident.

Men with sleep apnoea are more likely to have high blood pressure, cardiovascular disease (they're more likely to have a stroke) and ischemic heart disease (they're more prone to a heart attack).

Some men's snoring is caused by old sports injuries or accidents. If you broke your nose years ago, you could still have an obstructed nostril or deviated nasal septum — that's the bit in the middle of the nose dividing the nose into the left and right nostrils.

A bulky soft palate or a big tongue that falls back can also cause snoring, as can an unusually thick nose lining. Large tonsils are the commonest cause of snoring in boys.

Men with a fat neck are also more liable to snore. Fat is deposited and settles on the walls of the upper airways. This reduces the size of the air passages, making snoring more likely.

Treatments for Snoring

Men who sleep on their back are more likely to snore. They could try wearing a T-shirt backwards, with a golf ball or tennis ball in the pocket — to stop them rolling on to their back while asleep. Often, all a man has to do to stop snoring is to reduce his weight (Chapter 5). Temporary bouts of snoring can be due to a cold or flu or to allergies to pollen or dust. If you treat the cold or allergy, the snoring can cease or be reduced. You could also try breathe-easy nasal strips available from pharmacies.

Men who drink a lot are also more likely to snore. The solution is to drink less and earlier in the evening. Drinking earlier — or not at all — will also help you to get a better night's sleep.

If snoring persists and it's driving your partner demented or to the divorce courts, visit your GP, who may refer you to an ear, nose and throat (ENT) specialist with an interest in snoring or to a sleep laboratory.

Surgical options include laser assisted uvulopalatoplasty (LAUP). Dr Crowe warns: this treatment is 'very painful, absolutely. There's no saying that it isn't.' It will only be used if sleep is severely disrupted. You cannot avail of LAUP if you have sleep apnoea.

Continuous positive airway pressure (CPAP) may be offered to sleep apnoea patients. It's a machine which blows air through a nose mask into the upper airway at a designated pressure, depending on the individual patient. It acts like a pneumatic splint — the column of air keeps the passageway open. It can be rented or purchased. It's worn all night, every night and, yes, it's sexier than snoring.

Jaw replacement surgery may be offered to men whose snoring is caused by the tongue rolling back — but this surgery isn't widely available. Dental appliances are also available to help men with a posterially placed jaw.

CHAPTER 21

Men: Hair and Baldness

My problem is not changing my hair. It's keeping it,' said British Prime Minister Tony Blair, tongue-in-cheek, when responding to media suggestions that he had adopted the Caesar cut to attract women voters.

But many men don't find hair loss a laughing matter. Indeed, some men are obsessed with their balding pates. You would be unwise to argue with them that there are more important things in the world. Forever fixed in their uninsulated brain is their increasingly naked scalp.

It can be hard to stand up, just as you are, bald and proud. Yet the essence of manhood is surely something close to that — self-acceptance of ourselves and others just as we are and metaphorically and actually standing up, precisely as we are, maimed or bald and all.

Tinsel cut-outs of beautiful manhood, perpetuated by advertising and Hollywood, bamboozle us with images of the so called 'perfect' man. Admittedly, Hollywood didn't start it. The Bible presents the handsome Absalom as so hairy a specimen that his divested crop after each trip to the barber's weighed two hundred shekels — the weight of a few cans of beer.

It's a pity that some men feel the need to conceal their distinctiveness, and present a fake, time-warped self to the world, especially given the popularity of baldies like Sean Connery. Men don't need to hide behind the smoke-screen of artificial, or medically preserved, hair. It's not hair loss but the attempt to disguise the natural process of male pattern baldness that opens men up to ridicule. Just think of the wink and elbow tittering which can follow the sight of a middle-aged man, who should know better, wearing a ridiculous, ill-fitting hair-piece.

What is the price of vanity? The question was put by Dr Ronald Trancik of Clinical Research in Consumer Healthcare with Pharmacia & Upjohn in the United States. When speaking to Dr Trancik, a month's supply of the across-the-counter hair maintenance product, Regaine, cost £25.41. Someone who begins to use it at the age of 20 and goes on using it until his seventieth birthday, would spend £15,246.00 on the product, excluding price rises and inflation.

If you're willing to pay out that kind of money on preserving what hair you've got, you might consider using a fraction of it on a shrink and dealing with your self-esteem.

Dr Trancik admitted that this was a huge financial commitment 'on the man's part and on the part of the partner'. (How's that for a handicap to getting hitched? 'There's something I must tell you before we get to know one another better. I've got this financial commitment to my hair.')

Dr David Fenton, dermatologist with the Hair Clinic at St John's Institute of Dermatology, St Thomas's Hospital, London, feels that Regaine will not achieve dramatic results. It works best on men in their 20s or 30s and on those who have been balding for a short period. If you stop using the product, 'you lose it more quickly than you gained it'.

Dr Fenton believes that if you forestall baldness by ten years, your scalp will make up for lost time, perhaps within five years, relatively quickly arriving at the degree of baldness you would have reached if you hadn't interrupted male pattern baldness in the first place. But if this is the case, would it not be better to face the fear of gradual male pattern baldness now than in the throes of an accelerated loss in the event of stopping treatment later on? Do men really want to become so dependent on commercial products for their self-esteem?

Mr Niall Kiely, manager of Consumer Care at Pharmacia & Upjohn in Ireland, disagrees with Dr Fenton that the scalp makes up for lost time if you stop the treatment. He believes that if you stop treatment you proceed with male pattern baldness at your normal rate. On this question, Dr Trancik feels it is 'difficult to say', adding that subjects who took part in two year trials 'lost whatever they'd gained within six months'.

Male pattern baldness or androgenic alopecia accounts for about 95 per cent of balding heads. The process has already begun in earnest in as many as five per cent of 20-year-old men. Young men losing their hair should consider how distinctive they can look — and bear in mind the number of men who cut their hair tightly or shave it off altogether to enhance their appearance. Remember, too, being thin on top could help, rather than hinder, your search for the partner who is right for you.

Alopecia areata describes a condition of patchy baldness. Its cause is unknown and usually clears up completely within six to twelve months without treatment. Alopecia totalis is the rare loss of all scalp hair. When all bodily hairs fall out, the condition is called alopecia universalis. Traction alopecia is caused by rough brushing, aggressive towelling or ponytails, while localised friction alopecia is caused by wearing tight caps.

Hair and Cancer Treatments

When men have chemotherapy, they can lose their hair — but hair regrows fully after treatment has ended. Cooling the scalp with an ice-pack can protect the hair in some cases. When hair regrows, it can be thinner, curlier and of a slightly different colour than before.

Men who receive radiotherapy will lose hair only around the area being treated. It usually regrows completely after treatment, although its loss can sometimes be permanent. If and when it regrows, it tends to be thinner than before.

CHAPTER 22

Men: Teeth and Bad Breath

Men's teeth would appear to be in a healthier state than women's. Research conducted by Professor Denis O'Mullane, head of the University Dental School and Hospital in Cork, found that men had more teeth than women in every age group.

For instance, nearly a quarter of men aged 35 to 44 had 18 or more sound and untreated teeth (a full complement is 32) compared to only 13 per cent of women. In the 45 to 54 age bracket, 13 per cent of men retained 18 or more sound and untreated teeth, compared to only five per cent of women.

But if gender is a factor in the retention of teeth, so too is wealth — almost half of poorer men over 64 years of age had lost all their teeth, compared to only 17 per cent of men in higher income groups of the same age.

Why is it that men seem to do better than women in retaining their teeth? Men seem more willing to retain unattractive teeth while women tend to have them extracted for cosmetic purposes. The survey showed that men had higher tartar or calculus than women, indicating infrequent visits to the dentist.

Another possible reason why men have more teeth than women is, ironically, that women visit the dentist more often than men. Men are more likely to skip the recommended six monthly check-ups and only make it to the dentist when they can no longer bear a toothache.

Some well-meaning dentists in the past did harm as well as good by drilling and filling at the first sight of even slight tooth decay. But drilling weakens teeth because it involves digging deeper into the enamel. Dentists nowadays don't — or shouldn't — drill unless they have to.

In the past, they were only doing what scientists advised — and, often, what patients demanded. For instance, in the 1940s, many brides-to-be in Ireland and Britain had all their teeth extracted and dentures fitted as part of their marriage dowry.

But — and this is crucial — we now realise that dental decay can stop and heal up. When a person improves his oral hygiene and avoids sugar-grazing between meals, damaged enamel can re-mineralise and repair itself. If in the past the theory was, 'If in doubt, drill and fill', now it is (or should be) 'If in doubt, leave well-enough alone.' Be impressed with your dentist if he tells you there's slight decay, proposes a more rigorous oral hygiene routine, no sugar between meals, a check-up in six months and no fillings.

Be warned too: men who change their dentist end up with more fillings. It seems dentists recognise and trust their own work but often have niggling doubts about the work of their colleagues. This is understandable. They don't want a new patient to complain a week after a check-up that an old filling fell out and say that the new dentist should have spotted it.

It is also true that dentistry is not a precise science. In the 1980s, a British study found that 15 dentists presented with the same 18 patients made combined recommendations ranging from as low as only 20 fillings or replacement fillings to as many as 153. So never feel bad about seeking a second opinion if a dentist's proposed course of treatment involves lots of fillings. Simply tell him politely you would like to think about it, and get a second opinion.

Only 30 years ago, most 40-year olds had false teeth or were about to get them. Nowadays, so long as you eat sensibly and clean properly, you can expect to keep your teeth for life.

Young males should know that most tooth decay occurs before they are 20 years of age. During the ten or fifteen years after baby teeth fall out, people tend to do more damage to their teeth than during the whole of the rest of their lives. Elderly men who develop a sweet tooth late in life can also suffer a renewed acceleration of tooth decay.

No doubt you know that sugar is bad for your teeth. But the timing of sugar intake is also important. Sugar combines with mouth bacteria to launch an acid-attack on your teeth. The attack peaks 20 minutes after sugar intake and lingers for 30 minutes afterwards.

If you 'sugar-graze' between meals, you begin another 50 minute acid-attack before your teeth have had the chance to recover from your last meal. If you must take sugary snacks — most of which are not recommended because the saturated fat in them is also bad for your heart (see Chapter 4) — confine them to meal times. Eat fruit or bread at your 11 and 4 o'clock break. Fruit will do your teeth, heart, weight, energy levels and wallet (in the short term and long term) a big favour.

Incidentally, toothpaste sandwiches are bad for you. Regardless of what you see on the TV ads, you should only use a pea-sized portion of toothpaste. Dads, make sure your children don't use too much either, and they must not swallow it. Too much toothpaste can damage and blacken their teeth. Supervise your children's brushing and flossing until they are 7 years of age.

There is a debate about whether fluoride should or should not be put into the public water supply. In the main, fluoride is added to Ireland's water supply, while this is generally not done in Britain. As a result, some dentists say British and Irish teeth are radically different. They believe fluoride in more than 70 per cent of the Republic's public water supply has played a major role in improving the dental health of the nation. But environmentalists object to this, regarding fluoride as a toxic and corrosive poison.

If you live in an area which does not have fluoride in the public water system, some dentists argue that it's particularly important to use a toothpaste with fluoride. Professor Denis O'Mullane says that fluorideless toothpaste has little effect in preventing dental decay, although it does help to prevent gum disease. He questions the benefit of mouth-rinses and says that a nice taste does not mean a healthy mouth. Children under 7 shouldn't use mouth washes because they easily swallow them, he says.

Men and Trauma to the Teeth

Men are more prone to trauma of the front teeth than women, says Dr Jane Renehan, lecturer in public dental health at the Dublin Dental School and Hospital. She advises men engaged in contact sports to get a prescription gum shield made for their teeth. This costs a nominal sum but it could save a fortune in dental bills. Prevention is cheaper and better than cure.

If you have a tooth knocked out, for instance while playing sport, find the tooth, hold it by the crown (not the root) and rinse it in lukewarm water or milk. Do not clean the tooth with disinfectant. Replace it in the cavity — making sure you get it the right way up and not back-to-front. If you can't manage this, put the tooth in room temperature milk where it will live for up to four hours, or keep it in your mouth where it will live for two hours, and get yourself to a dentist fast.

Bad Breath

Halitosis, or bad breath, is usually caused by gum disease, so the first thing to do if you have bad breath is to see the dentist. An open cavity, a leaking filling or a loose crown or bridge can cause halitosis because of bacteria living in such places. But sometimes all that needs to be done is to have your teeth cleaned, scaled and the tartar removed.

Saliva breaks down bad breath. If you have bad breath in the morning, it could simply be because you produce less saliva at night. While you're asleep, fur gathers in the mouth which, when broken down by bacteria in the mouth, can cause a foul smell. Brushing your teeth and tongue after breakfast should disperse the bad odour in healthy mouths.

Eating sugar-free foods like fruit and vegetables regularly during the day stimulates saliva production and keeps breath fresh. Sipping water is good too because it keeps the mouth moist.

Garlic (although otherwise good for you), onions, curries and spicy foods emit foul-smelling chemicals from the lungs. Bad breath can also be due to alcohol fermentation in the stomach. However, parsley can neutralise the odour.

Halitosis can also be caused by smoking, tonsillitis, a large polyp or tumour in the sinuses, mouth cancer, chronic acidity or a hiatus hernia — that's when a part of the stomach protrudes upwards through the diaphragm. Other causes include a peptic ulcer, uncontrolled diabetes and diseases of the lung, liver, kidney or gall bladder.

CHAPTER 23

Men: Acne Versus that Porcelain Look

Men with acne can feel they're advertising disease on their face 24 hours a day. Little wonder, then, that men have committed suicide and others have become agoraphobic, withdrawing into themselves, and terrified even to go out, defeated by the psychological and social consequences that can accompany this disease.

Acne can deplete a man's quality of life. Studies have shown that adolescent males with acne tend to get depressed. They tend to do less well in exams than their porcelain-skinned peers. Men in their 20s, 30s and 40s with severe acne are discriminated against at job interviews, and they are more likely to be unemployed than their clear-skinned competitors.

Sexually, men with acne can feel less attractive. Men who do not freely choose celibacy can feel it is forced upon them because of their skin. They can fear that if the woman of their dreams unbuttoned their shirt, she might recoil at their spotty chest or back.

Acne can make it more difficult for men to find, and to enjoy the search, for a partner. It can diminish the joy of dating. It can hinder men from finding a partner and deprive them of the spiritual sustenance, growth and healing that can accompany a healthy, intimate relationship.

Acne can wreak havoc with a man's self-esteem. It can be difficult to feel good about yourself when a look in the mirror shows yet another wave of acne. It can be war wearying in its chronic persistence. No sooner has one cycle puckered and pounded your skin than another round begins. It can feel like there's no private space where you can escape the public gaze to soothe your sores and nurse your wounded pride. The battle is fought in public big time.

'Patients can have acne for four or five years and wonder will it ever end,' says consultant dermatologist Dr Bart Ramsay. He agrees that acne can impede men's formation of relationships, thwart their careers and reduce career options. He knows men who have given up a sport they love because they feel embarrassed by their naked lesion-covered back in the changing rooms.

Acne can have an effect on body fat, Dr Ramsay says. In men it reduces body fat, while women with acne have a tendency to gain weight. He says it's a myth that drinking lots of water, diet or facials help acne.

How Many Men Get Acne?

Up to 80 per cent of adolescent males get acne — just when young men are grappling with the messy business of growing up and when self-esteem and confidence can be at its most vulnerable.

Acne persists through the 20s, 30s, and even into the 40s, in up to five per cent of men. It can also start for the first time in older men.

Acne Vulgaris

Men tend to suffer from more severe acne than women. This is because acne vulgaris — the common acne which mainly afflicts adolescents and young adults — is caused by testosterone, the androgenic or male hormone. Hormonal changes can over-stimulate the production of sebum, the oil produced by the sebaceous glands in the skin. The excess of oil blocks the sebaceous glands, causing blackheads to appear. Bacteria living deep in the sebaceous glands now get to work. They break down the oil into fatty acids which seep into the surrounding skin, which goes red and a pimple or pustule appears.

Diet, Cleanliness and Acne

Many people are of the view that there is a connection between acne and the consumption of things like cream, chocolate, soft drinks and crisps. However, consultant dermatologist Dr Gillian Murphy says 'diet has nothing to do with acne'. She believes facial washes are a bit of a nonsense because acne vulgaris is not caused by dirty skin. In fact, men with acne are more likely to clean their skin more often than others. 'You don't get it from not washing,' she says.

Cystic Acne

Acne conglobata or cystic acne is a severe form of acne which affects more men than women. Abscesses and cysts can appear on the face, upper body, buttocks or legs, which can leave life-long scars.

Occupational Acne

Men whose skin is exposed to oil, tar or certain chemicals can be susceptible to developing occupational acne. Younger men who work in the fast food industry close to deep-fat fryers can also be at risk.

Cosmetic Acne

Men are less likely to develop cosmetic acne than women. But men who use cheap moisturisers, which can block skin ducts, can develop the condition.

Consultant dermatologist Dr Nicholas Walsh says older men have less acne than women and that this is possibly due to using fewer cosmetics than women.

Treatment

Men can feel, or be told, that they shouldn't be worried about a few spots or do anything about them because it's a bothersome phase they'll grow out of. Or, they might like to have the acne treated but feel they might be regarded as vain or unmanly for seeking treatment.

But men should seek treatment because acne can lead to life-long scarring. Dr Walsh says men should consult their GP and, if deemed necessary, see a dermatologist because, while the pimples will pass with time, the scars might not. Scars caused by acne can continue long after active acne has ceased. On this point, pimples and blackheads should not be squeezed as this can make scarring more likely.

Mild acne can be treated with benzoyl peroxide or topical antibiotics. Benzoyl peroxide, which is applied to the skin, can reduce acne by more than half within two months. It can be used in conjunction with certain kinds of topical antibiotics (that is, applied directly to the skin) and tretinoin (a topical cream or gel that speeds up the eruption of spots).

Moderate acne can be treated by applying azelaic acid, tretinoin or antibiotics like tetracycline. Antibiotics can also be taken in tablet form, for up to six months.

For severe acne, Roaccutane is seen as a wonder drug, says Dr Gillian Murphy. It can only be administered by a dermatologist and its possible side effects need to be carefully monitored.

There have been press reports linking Roaccutane to suicide but no definite causal link has been established — while the positive transformation in the skin, better looks and new confidence of men who use it is beyond doubt.

Useful Addresses

Addresses of organisations in both Ireland and the United Kingdom are provided below.

Ireland

Alcoholics Anonymous
109 South Circular Road, Leonard's Corner, Dublin 8.
Tel. 01 453 8998 *or* 01 679 5967 (after hours).

Aware — Helping to Defeat Depression
72 Lower Leeson Street, Dublin 2.
Tel. 01 661 7208. Helpline 01 676 6166.

Bereavement by Suicide
Northside Counselling Service, Coolock Development Centre,
Bunratty Drive, Bonnybrook, Dublin 17.
Tel. 01 848 4789 *or* Jean Casey 01 837 0433.

BODYWHYS (anorexia and bulimia nervosa)
P. O. Box 105, Blackrock, Co. Dublin.
Tel. 01 283 5126.

CÁIRDE (support for people with HIV and AIDS)
25 St Mary's Abbey (off Capel Street), Dublin 7.
Tel. 01 873 0800.

Clanwilliam Institute (personal, marriage and family therapy)
18 Clanwilliam Terrace, Grand Canal Quay, Dublin 2.
Tel. 01 676 1363 *or* 01 676 2881.

Dublin County Stress Clinic
St John of God Hospital, Stillorgan, Co. Dublin.
Tel. 01 288 1781.

Family Mediation Service (to help couples who have decided to
separate or divorce)
Block 1, Floor 5, Irish Life Centre, Lower Abbey Street, Dublin 1.
Tel. 01 872 8277.

Irish Cancer Society (variety of support groups)
5 Northumberland Road, Dublin 4.
Tel. 01 668 1855 *or* Freephone 1800 200 700.

Irish Family Planning Association (IFPA)
Unity Building, 16–17 Lower O'Connell Street, Dublin 1.
Tel. 01 878 0366.

Irish Heart Foundation
4 Clyde Road, Ballsbridge, Dublin 4.
Tel. 01 668 5001.

Irish Stillbirth and Neonatal Death Society (ISANDS)
Carmichael House, 4 North Brunswick Street, Dublin 7.
Tel. 01 872 6996 *or* 01 822 4688.

Irish Sudden Infant Death Association
Carmichael House, 4 North Brunswick Street, Dublin 7.
Tel. 01 873 2711 *or* 1850 391391 *or* 01 873 5702.

Men's Health

USEFUL ADDRESSES

Marriage and Relationship Counselling Services
24 Grafton Street, Dublin 2.
Tel. 01 679 9341 *or* 01 671 0902.

Men's Network
1 Silloge Road, Ballymun, Dublin 11.
Tel. 01 862 2194.

Parentline (helpline for parents)
Carmichael House, 4 North Brunswick Street, Dublin 7.
Tel. 01 873 3500 *or* 01 873 5702.

Parental Equality
1 Muirhevna, Dublin Road, Dundalk, Co. Louth.
Tel. 042 33163.

Samaritans
112 Marlborough Street, Dublin 1.
Tel. 01 872 7700 (24 hours a day) *or* 1850 60 90 90.

Separated Persons Association
Carmichael House, 4 North Brunswick Street, Dublin 7.
Tel. 01 872 0684 *or* 01 873 5702.

Rape Crisis Centre
70 Lower Leeson Street, Dublin 2.
Tel. 01 661 4911 *or* Freephone 1800 778 888.

Sleep Disorders Clinic
Mater Private Hospital, Eccles Street, Dublin 7.
Tel. 01 860 0090.

United Kingdom

Alcoholics Anonymous
P. O. Box 1, Stonebow House, Stonebow, York Y01 7NJ.
Tel. 01904 644026.

Anorexia and Bulimia Care
15 Fernhurst Gate, Ormskirk, Lancashire L39.
Tel. 01695 422479.

British Heart Foundation
14 Fitzhardinge Street, London W1H 4DH.
Tel. 0171 935 0185.

British Snoring and Sleep Apnoea Association
How Lane, Chipstead, Surrey CR5 3LT.
Tel. 01737 557997.

Cancer Aid and Listening Line
Swan Buildings, 20 Swan Street, Manchester M4 5JW.
Tel. 0161 835 2586.

CRUSE (bereavement helpline)
126 Sheen Road, Richmond, Surrey TW9 1UR.
Tel. 0181 940 4818.

CRY-SIS (for parents whose baby cries excessively)
BM Cry-sis, London WC1N 3XX.
Tel. 0171 404 5011.

Family Nurturing Network (parenting skills)
Unit 12F, Minns Estate, 7 West Way, Botley Road, Oxford
OX2 OJD.
Tel. 01865 722442.

Families Need Fathers
134 Curtain Road, London EC2A 3AR.
Tel. 0181 886 0970.

Family Planning Association
2–12 Pentonville Road, London N1 9FP.
Tel. 0171 837 5432. Helpline 0171 837 4044.

Impotence Association (advice and information)
P. O. Box 10296, London SW17 9WH.
Tel. 0181 767 7791.

MIND — National Association for Mental Health
15–19 Broadway, Stratford, London E15 4BQ.
Tel. 0181 519 2122.

National Family Mediation (for separating and divorcing couples)
9 Tavistock Place, London WC1H 9SN.
Tel. 0171 383 5993.

Parentline (support for distressed parents)
Endway House, The Endway, Hadleigh, Essex SS7 2AN.
Tel. 01702 559900 (24 hour helpline).

RELATE (relationship counselling)
Herbert Gray College, Little Church Street, Rugby CV21 3AP.
Tel. 01788 573241. Helpline 0870 601 2121.

SANELINE (emotional and crisis support)
1st Floor, Cityside House, 40 Adler Street, London E1 1EE.
Tel. 0345 678000.

Samaritans
10 The Grove, Slough, Berkshire.
Tel. 01753 532713; 0345 90 90 90.

Survivors (for men who have suffered sexual abuse or violence, either as children or in adulthood)
P. O. Box 2470, London SW9 9ZP.
Tel. 0171 833 3737.

Stillbirth and Neonatal Death Society (SANDS)
28 Portland Place, London W1N 4DE.
Tel. 0171 436 5881.

Further Reading

Banks, Dr Ian, *Ask Dr Ian About Men's Health*, Belfast: The Blackstaff Press 1997.

Brewer, Dr Sarah, *The Complete Book Of Men's Health*, London: Thorsons 1995.

Burgess, Adrienne, *Fatherhood Reclaimed*, London: Vermilion 1997.

Campbell, Joseph, *The Hero With A Thousand Faces*, London: HarperCollins 1988.

Carlson, Richard, *Don't Sweat The Small Stuff . . . And It's All Small Stuff*, London: Hodder & Stoughton 1998.

Cooper, Mick & Peter Baker, *The MANual: The Complete Man's Guide To Life*, London: Thorsons 1996.

Guinness, Louise (ed.) *Fathers: An Anthology*, London: Chatto & Windus 1996.

Hardiman, Michael, *Addiction: The CommonSense Approach*, Dublin: Newleaf 1998.

Huxley, Aldous, *The Perennial Philosophy*, London: Fontana 1966.

Hyde, Tom (ed.) *Fathers & Sons*, Dublin: Wolfhound Press 1995.

Jeffers, Susan, *Feel The Fear And Do It Anyway*, London: Rider 1991.

Kubler-Ross, Elisabeth, *On Death and Dying*, London: Routledge 1990.

Mark, Robert & Buddy Portugal, *Victories Of The Heart: The Inside Story Of A Pioneer Men's Group*, Rockport: Element Books 1996.

Mass, James B., *Miracle Sleep Cure: The Key To A Long Life Of Peak Performance*, London: Thorsons 1998.

Men's Health magazine, London: Rodale Press.

O'Hanlon, Brenda, *Sleep: The CommonSense Approach*, Dublin: Newleaf 1998.

O'Hanlon, Brenda, *Stress: The CommonSense Approach*, Dublin: Newleaf 1998.

Palmer, Helen, *The Enneagram: Understanding Yourself And The Others In Your Life*, San Francisco: HarperCollins 1991.

Real, Terrence, *I Don't Want to Talk About It: Overcoming the Secret Legacy of Male Depression*, Dublin: Newleaf 1998.

Sabo, Donald & Gordon David Frederick, *Men's Health And Illness: Gender, Power And The Body*, London: Sage Publications 1995.

Weatherill, Rob, *Cultural Collapse*, London: Free Association Books 1994.

Index